SECRETS TO HAPPINESS, INNER PEACE AND HEALTH

A Psychological, Spiritual and Physical Guide to Optimal Health and Fitness of the Body, Mind and Spirit.

By

Dr. Brian K. Bailey

© 1997

The health suggestions in this book are based on training, experience and research. It is meant to supplement and not replace your primary care physician. Please consult your doctor before making any significant dietary or exercise changes.

Copyright ©1997 Dr. Brian Keith Bailey

All rights reserved. No part of this book may be reproduced or transmitted in any form or by any means, electronic or mechanical, including photocopying, recording or by any information and retrieval system, without permission in writing by the author.

ISBN 0-9654904-0-8

$15.95 USA
$21.95 Canada

HEALTH UNLIMITED
1890 Waite St. Suite 6
North Bend, OR 97459
Printed in USA
First Edition

CONTENTS

ACKNOWLEDGMENTS

I thank God, for his unconditional love and guidance. I appreciate my guardian angels for always being there for me and helping me to find and follow my purpose. I am grateful for my mother, who taught be about unconditional love and helped me to develop self confidence and my dad for teaching me the principles of responsibility and persistence. Thank you Trisha for your 16 years of love and support. I thank Susan Smith Jones for fine tuning my skills as a writer and speaker, and for opening my eyes to the truth about health. I am grateful for my children Jeremy, Jared, Jonathan, Jennifer, Jeffery, Krystle and Kayla for their love. I pray that they will learn and understand the principles in this book. Last, but not least I cherish the love, support, understanding and editing by my best friend Sandra Whitney.

I thank Laura Nielsen, my good friend for her professional editing. Thank you Mardi Albright for your reading and editing.

My thanks to the following contributors:
Patty Wooten for *Humor the Healer*.
Susan Boyles for *Chakras*.
Charles R. Attwood, M.D. for *Milk, Calcium and Bone Density*.
Christian Hagaseth III. M.D. for the *12 Affirmations of Positive Humor*.

I give great thanks to the following authors for their knowledge and inspiration:
Dean Ornish, M.D., Julian Whitaker, M.D., Andrew Weil, M.D. John McDougal, M.D., Kenneth H. Cooper, M.D., Jean Carper, Deepak Chopra. M.D., Bernie Siegel, M. D., Larry Dossey, M.D., Norman Vincent Peale, Ph.D., John Gray, Ph.D., Barbara DeAngelis, Ph.D., Wayne Dyer, Ph.D., M. Scott Peck, M.D., Marianne Williamson, John Bradshaw, Ph.D., Herbert Benson, M. D., Dan Millman, Sir John Marks Templeton, Susan Smith Jones, Ph. D., Dale Carnegie, Larry King, Anthony Robbins. John

Robbins, Elson M Haas, M.D., Jack Canfield and Mark Victor Hansen, Pia Melody, Denis Waitley, John McDougal, M.D., Udo Erasmus, Edward N. Siguel, M.D., Ph.D., Gabriel Cousens, M.D., Kenneth H. Cooper, M.D., Melvin Morse, M.D., Pia Mellody, John-Roger and Peter McWilliams, Michael Newton, Ph.D.

PREFACE

In the process of looking for a publisher I consulted with a dozen literary agents. Their consensus was that this book should be split into two or more books, "you cover too many topics, why don't you expand your *12 Ways To Increase Your Metabolism* and make that a book?" While I have included everything you need to know to create the perfect body, that is not my purpose in writing this book. The reason I wrote this book was to put every aspect of health into one book. The body, mind and spirit are intimately connected, when one is not well the others suffer.

I first learned about physical health in school. This was my focus for over ten years of college, university and medical school training. Then, in the "school of life" I learned about the importance of emotional and spiritual wellness.

Gerald Kushel, EdD, was interviewed by the staff of *Bottom Line/Personal,*[1] (my favorite newsletter). He studied 1,200 people—lawyers, artists, blue collar workers, teachers and students. All of them seemed to have successful careers. What he found was:

- 15% did not enjoy their jobs or personal lives.
- 80% enjoyed their work but not their personal lives.
- 4% enjoyed both their work and their personal lives.

It is the purpose of the first half of this book to give you the emotional and spiritual skills to create happiness in your lives. I teach you how to find your purpose and set goals that are in alignment with your purpose. Someone once said that happiness is the gradual realization of a worthy goal.

Having studied the religions of the world, I have come to appreciate the beauty of each one as a tool for teaching spirituality. I reject the negative teachings of religion and embrace the positives. The greatest impact on my writing has come from many other great authors and speakers quoted throughout this book.[2] To the best of

---

[1] *Bottom Line / Personal* Sept. 15th 1996
[2] See the Suggested Reading at the end of the book.

my present ability, I have included all the major concepts necessary for us to increase our spirituality. I have written this book as much for me as I have for you.

Knowledge by itself is not enough, it takes constant practice here in our classroom, Earth. Pat Pearson once told a story about flying home from giving a speech; when the man sitting next to him learned he was a motivational speaker he said, "Aaah, that motivational stuff doesn't last. You get yourself all pumped up for a while and then it wears off." A passing flight attendant overheard him and said, "Well, a bath doesn't last either, but it's still a good idea." Pat goes on to say, "If you think about it, food doesn't last either. Exercise doesn't last. Everything in life needs to be renewed and nurtured, We feel hungry, we eat, we feel full, and in due time we get hungry again." This book is "manna," spiritual food. Eat some every day to nourish your spirit.

> *If there is light in the soul,*
> *There will be beauty in the person.*
> *If there is beauty in the person,*
> *There will be harmony in the home.*
> *If there is harmony in the home,*
> *There will be order in the nation.*
> *If there is order in the nation,*
> *There will be peace in the world.*
> —Chinese Proverb

You didn't think when you woke up this morning that this would be the day your life would change did you? But it's going to happen because the only thing that stands between you and grand success in living are these two things: Getting started and never quitting! You can solve your biggest problem by getting started, right here and now.
—Robert H. Schuller

PART ONE:

MENTAL, EMOTIONAL AND SPIRITUAL HEALTH

ATTITUDE

"We are all eagles, let go of our negative beliefs about ourselves and let's soar." Golden Eagle

The most remarkable transformations I have ever seen in a person have been due to a change in attitude. Everything about someone's life can change with their change of attitude. A positive, healthy attitude enables us to tap into the omnipotent and omniscient[1] strength within us.[2] We can become unlimited in our potential. Attitude is the essential key to true happiness, self esteem and the ability to give and receive love.

So, how do we develop a strong, healthy positive attitude? The first and most important principle to learn and incorporate into our daily lives is **acceptance.**

The central theme to acceptance is **understanding and accepting that life doesn't always** *seem* **fair**. We are unique. We all have different lessons to learn. When disappoinment happens ask yourself "what am I to learn from this experience?" Sometimes, we may not see the lesson right away. In order to see clearly we must get recentered.[3] Your Higher Power will light your path.[4] If we don't learn the lesson, the Teacher will keep giving it to us till we "get it."

Acceptance is recognizing that whatever happens in life and however we respond, is precisely what we need for our highest good and learning.

---

[1] Omnipotent is all powerful; omniscient is all knowing
[2] See the chapter: Angels, Guides and Guidance.
[3] See the chapter: Meditation.
[4] See the chapter: Angels, Guides and Guidance.

The second most important principle to learn is positive expectancy and positive self-talk. It is quite easy to say "Always expect good things and don't expect adversity." Well, as the bumper sticker says, "IT HAPPENS!" Adverse events temper our metal and can make us strong or destroy us depending on our attitude. Look at adversity as a challenge. The Chinese translate our word for crisis into two characters, the first character means dangerous, and the second means opportunity. Earl Nightingale once spoke of a business leader who, when told of an unfortunate event said, "That's good." He promptly looked for the good. It may take years of practice, affirmations and visualization to undo former negative thinking patterns.[5] Cancel both your negative thoughts and negative words. Whenever you say or think something negative, simply say **"cancel that"** and replace it with a positive thought or statement. For example, "This is going to be a rough day.....**cancel that**, today will be a challenging day, it will strengthen me." Here are some examples of positive versus negative traits:

1. Responsibility—We can choose to be empowered and responsible or we can choose to be a powerless victim. Victims appear stuck with whatever the world hands them. Generally, they get what they expect, more victimization. Empowered individuals choose to be responsible for everything in their lives, they are not blaming.

"Things turn out best for the people who make the best of the way things turn out"—John Wooden

2. Persistence, Determination—**and being a self starter** is the key to success and happiness. The quitter who is content with dependency on others will never find true happiness and fulfillment.

---

[5] See the chapters Visualization and Affirmations.

"Desire is the key to motivation, but it's the determination and commitment to an unrelenting pursuit of your goal—a commitment to excellence—that will enable you to attain the success you seek."
—Mario Andretti

"The difference between the impossible and the possible lies in a man's determination"
—Tommy Lasorda

3. Commitment—is the first step to achieving any goal. Commitment is the driving force over any obstacle. Lack of commitment leads to failure when the going gets tough.

"The quality of a person's life is in direct proportion to their commitment to excellence, regardless of their chosen field of endeavor."
—Vince T. Lombardi

4. Accomplishment—Be **proactive** versus **reactive.** The reactive person spends most of his time fixing or avoiding problems and never accomplishes much.

There are four steps to accomplishment:

1. Plan Purposefully.

2. Prepare Prayerfully.

3. Proceed Positively.

4. Pursue Persistently.

5. Adaptability—is what can keep you successful, being rigid and closed will cause you to meet the fate of the dinosaurs—extinction.

There is only one constant in life and that is change.

6. Opportunity—Remember to embrace opportunity and not to avoid and reject new situations.

Luck is talent meeting opportunity.

In the middle of every difficulty lies opportunity.

7. Perception—is everything, life is only what we perceive it to be. We can choose to believe that life is a beach and then we die, or we can believe that this minute, is the first minute, of the beginning of the rest of our wonderful lives. Alan Cohen writes about this in his book, *Joy is my Compass:* "the difference between a saint and a sourpuss is that the sourpuss sees his daily interactions as a nuisance, while the saint finds a continuous stream of opportunities to celebrate. One finds intruders, the other [finds] angels. At any given moment we have the power to choose what we will be and what we will see. Each of us has the ability to find holiness or attack about us."

"The pessimist sees difficulty in every opportunity. The optimist sees opportunity in every difficulty"
Winston Churchill

8. Enthusiasm—We can be enthusiastic or cynical, it is our choice. Enthusiasm is the propelling force necessary for climbing the ladder of success.

"You can't have rosy thoughts about the future when your mind is full of blues about the past"

9. Adversity—When life presents us with obstacles as it will, we can rise to the challenge and win or we can feel overwhelmed and lose.

> *If you can keep your head when all about you*
> *Are losing theirs and blaming it on you,*
> *If you can trust yourself when all men doubt you,*
> *But make allowance for their doubting too;*
> *If you can wait and not be tired by waiting,*
> *Or being lied about, don't deal in lies,*
> *Or being hated, don't give way to hating,*
> *And yet don't look too good, or talk too wise:*
> *If you can dream—and not make dreams your master;*
> *If you can think—and not make thoughts your aim;*
> *If you can meet with Triumph and Disaster*
> *And treat those two impostors just the same.*
> *if—*
> *If you can make one heap of all your winnings*
> *And risk it on one turn of pitch-and-toss,*
> *And lose, and start again at your beginnings*
> *And never breathe a word about your loss.*
> *If you can talk with crowds and keep your virtue,*
> *Or walk with Kings—nor lose the common touch,*
> *If neither foes nor loving friends can hurt you,*
> *If all men count with you, but none too much;*
> *If you can fill an unforgiving minute*
> *With sixty seconds worth of distance run,*
> *Yours is the Earth and everything that's in it,*
> *And—which is more—you'll be a Man, my son!*
> —Rudyard Kipling

Our attitude can be the anchor of the soul, the stimulus to action, and the incentive to achievement

10. Thankfuliving—If you are appreciative of what others do for you they will be much more likely to do more and work harder. If you are ungrateful or critical, people will try to avoid you.

John Marks Templeton in his book, *Discovering The Laws Of Life,* describes two women:

> "Two women work in the same office and receive the same pay. Anne complains that she is underpaid. She feels she's asked to handle too many things for someone on her salary level. She arrives dreading the day ahead and leaves tired and discouraged. Mary, on the other hand, is happy to have a secure job and enough money to pay her bills, with some left for extras and savings. She looks at each task as a challenge and does her best to accomplish whatever is demanded of her. She arrives looking forward to the day and leaves happy to be heading home to her family, feeling good about what she has accomplished. Not surprisingly, after an employee review, Mary receives both a promotion and a salary increase. Anne is let go."

Always have an attitude of gratitude

11. Love—We can choose to be either loving and caring or fearful and apathetic. In the book, *Love Is Letting Go Of Fear,* Gerald Jampolsky, M.D. says, "With love as our only reality, health and wholeness can be viewed as inner peace, and healing can be seen as letting go of fear. Love, then, is letting go of fear."

"The only thing we have to fear is fear itself"
Franklin D. Roosevelt

In my experience as a doctor, I have come to believe that physical illness is strongly tied to our emotional and spiritual health. The wholistic counseling I do proves this. Warm and tenderhearted people however, do get sick, because of other factors.[6] Dr. Hans Eysenck, a psychiatrist says that of all the risk factors that contribute to cancer, personality is one of the most important. Louise Hay, author of *Heal Yourself, Heal Your Life,* says "I find that resentment, criticism, guilt and fear cause the most problems in ourselves and our lives. Whatever is happening 'out there' is only a mirror of our own inner thinking."

12. Positive thinking[7]—Positive thinkers are curious, intrigued and constantly learning, always finding the good. Negative thinkers tend to be bored, critical and complaining.

The positive thinker sees the invisible, feels the intangible and achieves the impossible.

Positive people expect and create success, they work cooperatively with others and they are good team players. They are happy and hopeful regardless of their circumstances. Negative people usually expect and set up failure, they are dissenters and tend to isolate themselves from others. They are cynical and easily depressed.

"A person will be just about as happy as they make up their minds to be."
—Abraham Lincoln

13. Altruism[8]—and a sense of inter-connection with the world are qualities of a person with a positive attitude. Those with a negative attitude tend to be aloof and self-centered.

---

[6] See the physical health section.
[7] See the chapter: Belief: The Power of Positive Thinking.
[8] Good will, loving kindness or benevolence.

"This is the true joy in life, the being used for a purpose recognized by yourself as the mighty one; the being thoroughly worn out before you are thrown on the scrap heap; the being a force of nature instead of a feverish selfish little clod of ailments and grievances complaining that the world will not devote itself to making you happy. I am of the opinion that my life belongs to the whole community, and as long as I live it is my privilege to do for it whatever I can. I want to be thoroughly used up when I die. For the harder I work the more I live. I rejoice in life for its own sake. Life is no brief candle to me. It's a sort of splendid torch I've got to hold up for the moment and I want to make it burn as brightly as possible before handing it on to future generations. "—George Bernard Shaw

14. Honesty—and good character versus dishonesty and corruption.

"Sow an act, and you reap a habit, sow a habit, and you reap a character, sow a character and you reap a destiny"—Charles Reade

In *Hamlet*, William Shakespeare says: **"This above all: to thine own self be true, and it must follow, as the night the day, thou canst not then be false to any man."**

"The measure of a man's real character is what he would do if he would never be found out."
—Thomas MacCaullay

In the *Book Of Virtues*, by William J. Bennett, he writes:
Honesty expresses both self respect and respect for others.
Dishonesty fully respects neither oneself nor others. Honesty
imbues lives with openness, reliability and candor; it expresses
a disposition to live in the light. Dishonesty seeks shade, cover
or concealment. It is a disposition to live partly in the dark.

"Honesty is the first chapter in the book of wisdom."
—Thomas Jefferson

15. Creativity—versus destructiveness.

A creative attitude is the fuel of progress and growth.

16. Humor—sense of humor versus melancholy depression.[9]

17. Action oriented—a doer, a person that puts feet to their
dreams and prayers.

"Whatever you can do or dream you can, begin it, boldness has genius, power and magic in it"—Goethe

For about ten years, I have been subscribing to *Insight*. I receive
a monthly tape with messages on personal development. Brian
Tracy, the host, is one of my favorite speakers. Brian has
repeatedly emphasized four mental laws for personal achievement:

1. **Law of Belief.** This law states that whatever you believe with
    feeling, becomes your reality.[10]

---

[9] See the chapter: Humor: Jest for the Health of It.
[10] See the chapters: Belief: The Power Of Positive Thinking and Visualization.

2. **Law of Expectations.** This law states that whatever you expect with confidence, becomes your own self-fulfilling prophesy.
3. **Law of Attraction.** This law says that you are a "living magnet" and that you attract people and circumstances, ideas, opportunities, and resources necessary to help you achieve them.
4. **Law of Correspondence.** This law states that your outer world is a reflection of your inner world. Whatever it is you see in the world of people, places and things is a reflection of the inner attitude of your mind.

> *"The greatest revolution of my generation*
> *is the discovery that individuals, by*
> *changing their inner attitudes of mind,*
> *can change outer aspects of their lives."*
> —Dr. William James

18. Helping people become more positive thinkers.[11]
Millions of Americans have problems with depression, anger, anxiety, cynicism, pessimism, or the ability to express or feel positive emotions. Their negativity profoundly affects their performance, relationships, and the people around them. They get sick more often and affect the morale of everybody they come in contact with. Positivity can help turn them around. It can help the people near them cope more effectively. The minute they start to change so does their aura.[12] They go from growling to glowing. Stress, anxiety and anger begin to dissipate. As Henry Ford once said:

> *"Whether you think you can*
> *or think you can't, you are right."*

---

[11]See the chapter: Belief: The Power Of Positive Thinking.
[12] See the chapter: Chakras.

HUMILITY

"When you get cocky and start seeing things in black and white, Fate steps in and shakes things up a bit."
—Brad Pitt G.M.A. broadcast 9/21/95

When a patient praises me for my skills as a physician I **jokingly** say, "Thank you, I am good ... I am also proud of the fact that I am humble." What good is it to think you are humble and then think you are better than someone else that isn't humble?

Humility and pride are perhaps the most misunderstood concepts Jesus taught. There is nothing wrong with a strong positive self image. It is OK to believe you are good at your job or that you are a good parent. Being proud of oneself is no sin. It is when we start to believe that we are better than someone else because of our gifts from God that we err. As Jesus taught:

> *"Whoever exalts himself will be humbled and whoever humbles himself will be exalted"*
> —Matthew 23:12

It is a strange paradox. An old friend of mine once said, *"There is a God and I am not She."* Herein lies the secret to humility.

While we may posses personal power, that power comes from God. The more we think and behave as individuals, separate from all other beings and God, the more real power we lose. The greatest power that we can aspire for is *spiritual power.* This power is garnered though the realization of our interconnectedness to all beings, the earth, the universe and God.

> *"What shall it profit a man, if he shall gain the whole world, and lose his own soul"*
> —Mark 8:36

Humility is a primary requirement to fulfilling our purpose in life (to love unconditionally and to learn). We are not teachable unless we are humble. We will find loving others difficult, until we culture the humility inside ourselves.

Humility is simply being your authentic self, a child of God.

The quote that led me to my truest comprehension of humility is one by Dr. Walter Russell: **"Until one learns to lose oneself, he cannot find himself. The personal ego must be dissolved and replaced by the Universal ego."** My understanding of this was aided by John Marks Templeton's book, *Discovering the Laws of Life*. The ego is who we think we are—the physical self—achievements, career, family and possessions. It is this self that is competitive, feels hurt or angry if it doesn't get what it wants—**control**. The Universal self is the "higher self"—the spirit—a piece of the divine. Personal ego can blind us to the Universal ego within us just as the sun prevents us from seeing the stars in the daytime. Just as the sun goes down each day, we must dim our ego daily through meditation, to access the spirit within. The spirit has access to Universal knowledge.

John Marks Templeton says, "In being humble we discover that humility rewards itself. When we are willing to put aside the whims and demands of our personal selves to listen to the guidance of the greater self within, we will gain access to an infinite source of power. This universal ego is as much (perhaps more than) who we are as the personal ego. It is infinitely more loving and wise and is always there for us. The more we put aside what we ordinarily think of as ourselves and identify with our higher selves, the more we come to recognize that this is our real, essential self. When we are humble in this new identification we are able to produce far greater results than we dreamed possible, thus securing greatness through humility."

ACCEPTANCE

This could be titled *TRUST*, acceptance is trust of God or whatever you conceive as your higher power. Acceptance is a major key to peace, serenity and stress reduction. It is believing that everything that happens in life is for your best good. It is recognizing that whatever happens in life and however we respond, is precisely what we need for our highest good and learning.

Sometimes we lose sight of who we really are. **We are not human beings having a spiritual experience, we are spiritual beings having a human experience.** We must keep sight of our purpose in life; that is to grow spiritually.

Our experiences here are our teachers. To learn the most and avoid repeating our personal history, learn *to let go of control and let God*. Trying to control things or people will cause frustration and rob us our peace and serenity, our life will become unmanageable. **Whatever we try to control will end up controlling us.** The only thing we can control is our mind and that is not easy.[13] If you want to enjoy a peaceful happy life, find your purpose and plan the roadmap to fulfill it. When you believe you can control other people you must think you are more powerful than God.

One of my favorite prayers is the codependent's prayer:

God grant me the serenity to accept the people I cannot change.
The courage to change the person I can. And the wisdom to know it is me.

---

[13] See the chapter: Visualization.

"Life is difficult. This is a great truth, one of the greatest truths. It is a great truth because once we truly see this truth, we transcend it. Once we know that life is difficult—then life is no longer difficult. Because once it is accepted, the fact that life is difficult no longer matters."—M. Scott Peck from *The Road Less Traveled.*

Taking personal responsibility for our lives is essential to acceptance. **Realize: If it is to be it is up to me.** It is our responsibility to turn within to seek the help we need. Within us, is our spirit and that spirit has unlimited potential.[14]

A major road block to acceptance is **blame.** We may blame our parents, the government or anybody for whatever is going on in our lives. As long as we blame others, we give our personal power away. We no longer have power to change our lives if we blame others for our ruined life. If we truly want to live, we need to realize that we have the power to change. *We are the Captains of our souls, the masters of our destiny.* We may also blame the past and feel that we "have blown it." The past is history, learn from it, let it go and move on. *Have no <u>regrets</u> for your past, your past has shaped you into who you are.* Some people, particularly those in organized religion may blame demons or evil spirits for their actions. **Demons and evil spirits are the negative thoughts and emotions we carry and hold on to.** C. S. Lewis, a prominent Christian author believes in demons and devils. Even so, in his book *The Grand Miracle,*[15] he says, "No reference to the Devil or devils is included in any Christian Creeds."

*I accept full responsibility for my life
and I trust God that everything that
happens in my life is for my best good.*

---

[14] The spirit's unlimited potential will be covered in detail in later chapters.
[15] Chapter 3, question 9, page 31.

FINDING YOUR PURPOSE

A life without purpose is like a trip without direction.

Some people live their whole lives without purpose. When they approach the end of their sojourn on earth they fear death and think, is that all there is?

"Great minds have purposes, others have wishes."
—Washington Irving

Dr. Viktor Frankl, an Austrian psychologist who survived the death camps of Nazi Germany, made an important discovery. He found one factor above all others including—health, survival skills and intelligence. This factor was purpose—a future vision of work they were yet to do, a mission to perform. Dr. Frankl said we don't invent our mission; we detect it. It is within us waiting to be realized.

Everyone has a purpose, it is not a goal that can be attained, purpose is like a direction your life is headed.

My personal mission statement is:
To love and serve humankind by helping as many people as I can to be healthy: spiritually, emotionally and physically. To do this I will keep myself healthy: spiritually, emotionally and physically. I will follow the precepts in my book, *Secrets to Happiness, Inner Peace and Health* to the best of my ability. In order to serve well, I will constantly read, write, study and speak about all areas dealing with health of the body, mind and spirit. To improve my ability to serve my purpose, I will remember my humanity by helping people on a personal and individual basis. I will tithe my time, talents or resources to help those in need including worthy causes.

Creating your own empowering mission statement takes a very deep examination of who you are and why you are here. You will have the answers to these questions when you thoroughly understand the first half of this book. Your mission statement will use your talents, provide for personal growth in all ten areas listed for goal setting (next chapter) and have a transcendent purpose.[16] *Your personal mission statement is written to inspire you—not to impress anyone else.* Your mission was chosen by you before you came into your body, to this time and place. It is the reason you are here. It is why you are now reading this. **Fulfill your destiny.**

An important set of clues to your purpose are the talents you were given and the direction life has been trying to point you. Another clue is what do you do that gives you the most lasting pleasure. The reward of following your purpose is happiness and fulfillment. Do the best you can now to discover your purpose, schedule a personal retreat as close to nature as possible to refine it.

Have a picture in your mind of who you want to become to accomplish your mission. I have a picture in my mind of who I am becoming. My picture is a combination of many people most of whom I have quoted in this book.[17]

For someone to find their purpose, all they need to do is listen. Many people pray to find their answers but fail to listen. By sitting quietly, not thinking, just listening that the answers will come.[18] Part of our purpose here on earth is for advancement of our spirituality, which is a primary goal of this book. This book is designed to help you understand and learn from the school of life. The school of life will constantly give you learning situations necessary for your spiritual progression. Develop a constant awareness and search for meaning in life's events. There will be people, places and things that are "signposts" for which direction

---

[16] Transcendent purpose is a purpose higher than self.
[17] See Acknowledgments.
[18] See the Meditation and Visualization chapters.

your life is to head. More will be taught about this in later chapters.

What in the world would you like to see changed the most? This is a clue to your purpose. If you could do anything to help the world, what would it be? To help you answer this, list your talents. How can these talents assist the world in positive change? Are there talents you can develop or acquire that will help you?

Changing the world begins with changing yourself. The positive example that you give to a child may have more influence on the world than a lifetime career.[19]

The most important work you ever do may be within the four walls of your own home.

I have a purpose, if I listen quietly it will be revealed to me. I will be directed in my life everyday when I take the time to listen.

---

[19] You don't have to be a parent to influence children.

GOALS

"If you fail to plan you plan to fail"
Ben Franklin

While purpose is the direction your life is headed, goals are the destinations. Goals require a roadmap. Short term goals are where we plan to be each day on our trip through life. Long term goals are where we plan on being in future years. With no goals, or if we lose sight of our goals, we will lose our sense of direction or purpose.

"If you want to be happy, set a goal that commands your thoughts, liberates your energy and inspires your hopes."
Andrew Carnegie

First, set your long term goals. Dream big, have no limits—what would you do if you had no limits? Describe the steps necessary to get there. In order to track your progress, these steps must be measurable and have a time table for their accomplishment. Always make sure your goals are in alignment with your purpose and your life's mission statement.[20]

"Where there is no vision the people perish."
Proverbs 29:18

"Obstacles are those frightful things you see when you take your eyes off your goal."—Henry Ford

I am going to list 10 areas of personal growth, please rate each area from 1 to 10 with 5 being average and 10 perfect (based on your ideal of perfect for you eg. what you are happy with). Start

---

[20] See the chapter: Finding Your Purpose.

with five years ago, then today and end with where you want to be in five years:

	5yrs ago	Today	5yrs future
Physically	_______	_______	_______
Mentally	_______	_______	_______
Emotionally	_______	_______	_______
Spiritually	_______	_______	_______
Relationship	_______	_______	_______
Family	_______	_______	_______
Career	_______	_______	_______
Financially	_______	_______	_______
Living environment	_______	_______	_______
Socially	_______	_______	_______

Rank these areas on paper from 1 to 10 based on their importance to you (you may add other areas that are important to you). Now, on separate sheets of paper brainstorm for at least 5 minutes each on everything you would like to do to improve in each area. This brainstorming must be done without limits as to money, time or anything else. Write everything that comes to mind no matter how silly or impractical it seems at the moment. Now, review each area and pick one thing you can do immediately and rate at least 4 more that you will begin when the first one is done or being done. Make a commitment to accomplish goals in as many areas as you feel comfortable with now. Goals without commitment and persistence are worthless.

W.H. Murray, in *The Scottish Himalayan Expedition*, explained it thus:

> Until one is committed, there is hesitancy, the chance to draw back, always ineffectiveness. Concerning all acts of initiative (and creation) there is one elementary truth, the

ignorance of which kills countless ideas and splendid plans: that **the moment one definitely commits oneself, then Providence moves too.** All sorts of things occur to help one that would never other wise have occurred. A whole stream of events issues from the decision, raising in one's favor all manner of unforeseen incidents and meetings and material assistance, which no man could have dreamed would have come his way. I have learned a deep respect for one of Goethe's couplets:

> *Whatever you can do,*
> *or dream you can, begin it.*
> *Boldness has genius,*
> *power and magic in it.*

Once your goals are made, make your commitments, believe, visualize and affirm their fulfillment.

I challenge you, right now to quickly fill in the following form or copy it and place it on your bathroom mirror. This is the beginning of a new and more productive life. Later, you will want to spend more time and perfect these goals. For now, this gets you started. **No more procrastination!**

Set a Date—as John Marks Templeton said,[21] "A deadline is to a task what a corral is to a herd of wild horses. It surrounds untamed impressions, thoughts and feelings with a clear boundary which allows your ideas to formulate as an attainable goal. Most people cannot effectively begin a project until they can see an end to it, a point of fulfillment. **A goal without a deadline is a goal never reached.** ... Remember, deadlines are lifelines that define your unlimited success." Keep your deadline flexible so if unforeseen problems arise it can be reset.

---

[21] In his book Discovering the Laws of Life.

"If one advances confidently in the direction of his dreams, and endeavors to live the life which he has imagined, he will meet with a success unexpected in common hours... If you have built sandcastles in the air, your work need not be lost; that is where they should be. Now, put foundations under them."
—Henry David Thoreau

Goals

<u>date to begin/finish</u>

Physical:

Mental (continuing education)**:**

Emotional:

Spiritual:

Relationship:

Family:

Career:

Financial:

Living Environment:

Social (service to community)**:**

Six final rules:

1. Make sure your goals are in alignment with your personal mission statement.
2. Make your goals specific.
3. Set a deadline.
4. Write as much detail about your goals as possible.
5. Learn all you can about your goals.
6. Search diligently for opportunity, expect to find it.
7. Be persistent, work hard, enjoy the process.

Aim at the moon and you will never shoot yourself in the foot.

JOURNALING

If you want to be your own therapist, keep a journal.

Journaling is an excellent tool for tracking life's progress. It is also an excellent way to process each days events. A good way to start your day is to begin by reviewing your personal mission statement,[22] tracking the progress on reaching your goals,[23] reading your affirmations[24] and meditating.[25] A good way to end your day is to review your goals and journal your progress. This is also the best time to make your next day's goals. Periodically (monthly or quarterly) review and modify intermediate and short term goals.

Each day record:
- The lessons you learn.
- The good that you or others do.
- The significant events of the day and your feelings about them.
- The insights you have and how you will do things differently in the future.
- Visualize your future as you want it to be.[26]

In the beginning keep it simple and easy, make it fun. I used to tape record instead of write. There does seem to be something special about writing, it seems to tap into the deeper part of who you are, perhaps your spirit. If it seems too overwhelming to do it daily then pick a day and time to do it each week e.g. Sunday evening at 8 PM.

---

[22] See the chapter: Finding Your Purpose.
[23] See the chapter: Goals.
[24] See the chapter: Affirmations.
[25] See the chapter: Meditation.
[26] See the chapter: Visualization.

Research shows that talking with a close friend about your feelings or writing them down greatly relieves stress. You will find that reviewing your journal will reveal thought and behavior patterns—good ones and bad ones. You will see decisions and directions you've taken. Often you will realize that you will need to change certain patterns in order to enjoy a more happy, healthy life.

> *Review your journal with the eye*
> *that everything happens for a reason,*
> *to teach you something. Learn that lesson*
> *so you won't need to repeat it again.*

CHANGE

*"You are not being called upon to change yourself.
You are being asked to be more of what you already
are. The invitation is bold, the stakes are high, and the
outcome certain. Dare to live your destiny now."*
—Alan Cohen

There is only one constant or sure thing in life and that is change. The world is constantly changing.

Many people live their lives doing the same old things in the same old ways. They refuse to leave their comfort zone of habit. They who lack the courage to step out and try new things are damned to progression and learning. It is boring to spend time with them. I find it exciting and interesting to be with someone who is forever trying new methods and ideas. I learned a very valuable adage in medical school when talking about new drugs, "Never be the first to change nor the last."

This is where intuition becomes invaluable. Listen to that small, still voice inside to know when to make changes. Sometimes, it may tell you to go against conventional wisdom and be the first to change.

*"Man is made or unmade by himself.
By the right choice he ascends.
As a being of power, intelligence and love
and lord of his own thoughts,
he holds the key to every situation."*
—James Allen

I heard a great story once that helped me understand personal change.[27] The story was about Michelangelo and his creation of the statue of David.

Several hundred years ago a rich and powerful family in Florence, Italy commissioned Michelangelo to create a statue for the main square.

Michelangelo spent two years searching for the right piece of stone to create his masterpiece. To his surprise one day he noticed a stone covered with weeds and dirt on a street he had walked past several times. He studied the stone and in it he saw clearly the statue of David. He had workmen deliver the stone to his studio. He began the hard long task of hammering and chiseling. It took him two years to produce a rough outline of the statue. He then put away the hammers and chisels and spent two more years of sanding and polishing. A crowd of thousands came to the unveiling, when they saw the statue of David, they were awestruck. It was clearly the finest work they had ever seen.

Later, Michelangelo was asked how he was able to create such a masterpiece, he simply said that he saw the David in the marble and he simply removed all the stone that was not the David.

As for my life, it took me years to find I was trapped in stone. I wanted out yesterday. It took years to chip away all that was not me. It will take many more years to finish the sanding and polishing. While we can make dramatic changes in a short time, it will take years, perhaps a life time to finish the polishing. Begin it today and use this book as your road map.

I WILL BE COURAGEOUS ENOUGH TO STEP OUT OF MY COMFORT ZONE AND TRY NEW THINGS.

---

[27] Insight tape #164, Nightingale-Conant Corp. 1-800-323-5552.

SUCCESS

*"Never lose sight of the fact that
the most important yardstick of your success will be how
you treat other people—your family, friends &
coworkers and even strangers you meet along the way."*
—Barbara Bush

In my study of successful people, I have found many common characteristics, perhaps the most powerful ones are: **PERSISTENCE coupled with DETERMINATION.**

*"**NOTHING IN THE WORLD CAN TAKE THE
PLACE OF PERSISTENCE. TALENT WILL
NOT : NOTHING IS MORE COMMON THAN
UNSUCCESSFUL MEN WITH TALENT.
GENIUS WILL NOT : UNREWARDED
GENIUS IS ALMOST A PROVERB
EDUCATION ALONE WILL NOT : THE
WORLD IS FULL OF EDUCATED DERELICTS.
PERSISTENCE AND DETERMINATION
ALONE ARE OMNIPOTENT.**"*
—Calvin Coolidge

One important point that must be remembered, is that you can have anything you want, but you can't have everything.[28] When you choose your goals and path in life there will be sacrifices. For example, if you want to be an Olympic athlete there will be very little room for other activities for years. Most of your life will be spent training or resting for the next workout.

Read the biographies of the people you would like to emulate. In most biographies, you will find a long hard road paved with

---

[28] Oprah Winfrey says that you can have everything, just not everything at the same time.

failure and disappointment. These lessons were necessary to show the path to success. Like the refiner's fire produces quality metal and the trial of fire, ice and folding of metal produces a fine sword.

Albert Einstein didn't speak until age four and didn't read until age seven. His teacher described him as, "mentally slow, unsociable and adrift forever in his foolish dreams." He was expelled and refused admittance to the Zurich Polytechnic School.

Walt Disney was fired for lack of ideas by a newspaper editor. He also went bankrupt several times before he built Disneyland. Henry Ford went broke five times before he finally succeeded. Babe Ruth holds the record for being struckout. Thomas Edison's teacher said he was too stupid to learn anything. You can read 18 more similar stories in the *New York Times,* #1 bestseller, *Chicken Soup for the Soul* and 48 more in its two sequels, both *New York Times,* #1 bestsellers. In the *3rd Serving of Chicken Soup for the Soul,* Jack Canfield and Mark Victor Hansen write:

- When we wrote *Chicken Soup for the Soul,* it was turned down by 33 publishers before Health Communications agreed to publish it. All the major New York publishers said, "it is too nicey-nice" and "Nobody wants to read a book of short little stories." Since that time over 7 million copies of *Chicken Soup for the Soul, A 2nd Helping of Chicken Soup for the Soul* and the *Chicken Soup for the Soul Cookbook* have been sold worldwide, with these books translated into 20 languages.

The life of Abraham Lincoln is probably the greatest example of persistence:

1816	His family was forced out of their home He had to work to support them.
1818	Death of his mother and sister as a child Entered the Blackhawk War as a captain by the end of the war demoted to private.
1831	Failed business partnership in a general store

1832   Defeat as a candidate for state legislature.
       Also lost his job—he couldn't get into law school
1833   Borrowed money from a friend to begin a business and
       by the end of the year he was bankrupt.
1835   Death of his sweetheart.
1836   Suffered a nervous breakdown and was bed ridden for 6
       months.
Death of three of his young sons.
1843 and 1844, Defeat when he ran for congress.
1849   Lost nomination as commissioner
1855   Defeat as a candidate for Senate.
1856   Defeat as vice presidential candidate.
1858   Defeat as a candidate for Senate.

Even as president he had his detractors. Here is a letter he wrote as president:

"If I were trying to read, much less answer, all the attacks made on me, this shop might well be closed for any other business. I do the best I know how, the very best I can; and I mean to keep on doing it to the end. If the end brings me out all right, what is said against me will not amount to anything. If the end brings me out all wrong, ten angels swearing I was right would make no difference."

This quotation was given to Winston Churchill on his 70th birthday by Franklin Delano Roosevelt. It became one of his favorite quotes. Churchill failed the 6th grade.

"Never, Never, Never Quit." Winston Churchill

"Far better it is to dare mighty things, to win glorious triumphs even though checkered by failure, than to rank with those poor spirits who neither enjoy nor suffer much because they live in the gray twilight that knows neither victory nor defeat."
—Theodore Roosevelt

Don't Quit

When things go wrong as they sometimes will.
When the road your trudging seems all up hill.
When funds are low and debts are high.
And you want to smile, but you have to sigh.
When care is pressing you down a bit.
Life is queer with its twists and turns.
As everyone of us sometimes learns.
And many a failure turns about.
When he might have won had he stuck it out:
Don't give up though the pace seems slow—
You may succeed with another blow.
Success is failure turned inside out—
The silver tint of the clouds of doubt.
And you can never tell how close you are.
It may be near when it seems so far:
So stick to the fight when you are hardest hit—
It's when things seem worst that you must not QUIT.

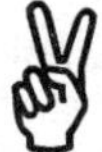

Author unknown

Persistence is one essential quality to success, however, without a plan or a path it is worthless. Life is very much like a journey. We need to know where we are going and have a road map of how to get there.

> ***"Those who fail to plan, plan to fail."***
> Ben Franklin

The very first step is to determine what we want in life. What would you do if you had no limitations? What are the sacrifices involved? Am I willing to make the sacrifices? Make your plan, set your goals and write your road map.

THERE IS NOTHING TO IT BUT TO DO IT!

What stops us from achieving our goals? **FEAR of FAILURE** stops us from beginning. Lack of **commitment, disipline or clear vision** will allow us to quit. ***Put feet to your prayers. Plan your work and work your plan.***

> ***SOMEDAY ISLE*** *IS A PLACE SOME PEOPLE SPEND THEIR LIVES, If you want to make changes in your life <u>do it now</u> or set a date.*

Remember to be flexible for the one constant in life is change. The roadmap you have made is much like that of a pilot's. There are constantly changing crosswinds and the pilot must continually make course corrections. If you are not making course corrections you may arrive in a totally different place than you expected.

> ***"Use wisely your power of choice."***
> Og Mandino

The **greatest power** we have is the **power of choice**. Life is all a choice. We can choose everything we do. We are right now, the sum total of all our past life choices. Don't give that power away. If you have, like many others, then, reclaim it!

There is **nothing** we have to do. When we say I have to do this or that, we then become slaves to whatever it is we have to do. Don't say **have to** instead say **choose to**. Other words to eliminate are negative or limiting words such as:

HAVE TO	**SHOULD**	**INADEQUATE**
HATE	**TRY**	**IMPOSSIBLE**
OUGHT TO	**CAN'T**	**LIMITATION**
NEVER	**ALWAYS**	**DIFFICULT**
BUT	**DOUBT**	**HOPELESS**
IF ONLY	**FAILURE**	**MAKES ME FEEL**

"To laugh often and much; to win the respect of intelligent people and the affection of children; to earn the appreciation of honest critics and endure the betrayal of false friends; to appreciate beauty; to find the best in others; to leave the world a bit better, whether by a healthy child, a garden patch or a redeemed social condition; to know even one life has breathed easier because you have lived. This is to have succeeded."
—Ralph Waldo Emerson

♥ I am responsible for my success. ♥

RESPONSIBILITY

(RESPONSE-ABILITY)

"THE PRICE OF GREATNESS IS RESPONSIBILITY."

WINSTON CHURCHILL

The most important characteristic of the spiritually mature individual is responsibility. A spiritually mature person takes responsibility for everything they have created in their life. They accept their life as it is and blame no person, place or thing for their circumstances. They will admit when they make a mistake without excuses, they apologize.

Those who fail to take responsibility for and learn from their mistakes are condemned to repeat them.

If you don't take responsibility for a mistake there is no reason to learn from it, because, after all it was not your fault.

Being responsible means getting organized, disciplined and developing a plan for your life. The responsible person develops self control and channels their energies into endeavors that will best serve them and the world.

Enjoy your daily work and do it joyfully.

Realize: If it is to be it is up to me.

MISTAKES

"Aim for success, not perfection. Never give up your right to be wrong, because then you will lose the ability to learn new things and move forward in your life. Remember that fear always lurks behind perfectionism. Confronting your fears and allowing yourself the right to be human can, paradoxically, make you a far happier and more productive person."
—Dr. David M. Burns

Our best lessons in life are taught to us through mistakes. Mistakes help us grow in character and spirituality. Some people spend their lives trying to avoid situations that may cause them to fail. They are not living their lives fully. The majority of successful people have made numerous mistakes. In movie making, if the scene isn't quite right it is a mis-take and it is repeated until it is right. Every mistake has a lesson to learn, if we fail to learn the lesson, we will likely repeat the mistake.

Insanity is when we do the same thing over again and expect different results.

We can only learn from mistakes if we admit to them, take responsibility and own them. Admit your mistake, don't make excuses—apologize.

"Character cannot be developed in ease and quiet. Only through experiences of trial and suffering can the soul be strengthened, vision cleared, ambition inspired and success achieved."
—Helen Keller

> ***"A man can fail many times but he isn't a failure until he begins to blame others."***
> —Ted Engstrom

It is easier to blame our teacher for our difficulties than to take the responsibility ourselves. Have you ever taught a person to ride a bike or roller skate? When they fall, do they blame their own inexperience or do they say, "It was your fault for letting go too soon or holding on too long"? How often do you hear, "They made me do it"? It is so easy to think that someone or something makes us fail. The powerful response is to be responsible for your own life. Don't give your power, and your future away. Remember to be gentle with yourself.

> **"WE LEARN WISDOM FROM FAILURE MUCH MORE THAN FROM SUCCESS; WE OFTEN DISCOVER WHAT WILL DO, by finding out what will not do; and probably he who never made a mistake never made a discovery."**
> —Samuel Smiles

When a friend is fretting over a mistake, say, **"Guess what, you're human."** When I make a mistake and start to "beat myself up" I remind myself there is a God and I am not He. Always forgive yourself and accept God's forgiveness. Remember:

> **We are children of God and are loved, not for what we have or do, we are loved just because we Are.**

You are not your performance. Be gentle with yourself, strive for excellence, not perfection.

*Don't sweat the small stuff and remember
everything is small stuff.*
—Anthony Robbins

Develop a good sense of humor and take life lightly.

We can't change the past, we can only rise above it. Learn from the past, plan for the future, and live fully in the present. Be grateful for the "hurts" you receive, for they are channels of understanding and wisdom. Be grateful for all the trials and tribulations in your life, for they are your teachers.

Have no <u>regrets</u> for your past, your past has shaped you into who you are.

An old African proverb teaches us to learn from our mistakes,

"Do not look where you fell, but where you slipped."

"While one person hesitates because he feels inferior, the other is busy making mistakes and becoming superior."
—Hugh Link

I WILL WELCOME MISTAKES IN MY LIFE AS AN OPPORTUNITY TO LEARN AND TO GROW SPIRITUALLY.

FORGIVENESS

*"To be wronged is nothing unless
you continue to remember it."*
—Confucius

We **all** carry baggage from our past experiences: blaming, regrets, pain, denial (of events or failure to grieve). **Baggage will sabotage your life, especially relationships**. Unresolved past events (things that were not and are not being worked on) will come out **sideways** and hurt those you love most. Baggage will weigh us down and prevent us from soaring to spiritual heights. **Let go! Forgive, grieve, accept your pain and your past mistakes.**

Blaming can often block us from further progression in our spiritual growth. If something that you perceive as **awful** has happened in your life replace blaming with acceptance and forgiveness. If you **blame the perpetrator** and say, "He or she has **ruined my life" then your spiritual growth is damned until you forgive this person and regain your personal power**. This long past event causes you to feel hurt and angry. The **anger can ultimately consume you with hatred**. This is your hatred. **You own it** and carry it around with you wherever you go. This power you have given away will sabotage all your relationships. **Let it go**, forgive and release the power of this past event. Move on with your life. Realize, **this next hour is the first hour of the rest of your life. You are the Master of your destiny, the Captain of your own soul.**

If you can feel it you can heal it

I have a very strong sense of justice, it is hard for me to **let go and let God**. However, as the Chinese proverb states: **"The one who pursues revenge should dig two graves."**

One of the keys to forgiving someone who has hurt you, is understanding them. What has their life been like? What influences shaped their behavior? When you understand your offender you will forgive them. Forgiveness does not mean excusing their offense; there is no excuse for abuse. Your job is to accept the past, be grateful for what you have learned from it and move on with your life. Karma[29] will provide the necessary lessons for those involved.

Another big part of forgiveness is **judgment**. The Bible tells us not to judge. Judgment is a part of life; everything we do is based on some type of judgment eg. between chocolate and vanilla or whatever. Since it is difficult not to judge, develop your **empathy**[30] for others. When we judge, we need to walk a mile or more in the shoes of whomever we are judging. If we practice acceptance (forgiveness in action) we avoid the hurt that goes with judging.

Some of us carry a tremendous burden. **That burden of unforgiveness can pile up to a point that causes physical disease.** Some doctors, myself included, believe that some autoimmune diseases, cancer, heart disease and arthritis are tied to negative emotional states. The most destructive emotional state is unresolved hurts. Search your heart and systematically accept, forgive and let go of past hurts.

> *"To err is human, to forgive divine."*
> —Alexander Pope

---

[29] Whatever we put into the world comes back to us.
[30] Empathy is genuine emotional and spiritual understanding.

Jest for the Health of It!
"HUMOR: THE HEALER"
based on an article by Patty Wooten, RN, BSN
used with permission.

Humor is a great stress reliever, it enables us to experience joy even when faced with adversity. Stress is the result of fear, it prepares our bodies to fight or run. The exercise of fighting or running lessens the negative effects on our bodies. However, in the modern world we can't always fight or run, but, we can laugh. The fears we feel are **often** not real, just phantoms from our past.[31] The fears we feel may also come from situations in which we feel out of control or don't understand the purpose of life.

Finding humor in a situation and laughing freely with others can be a powerful antidote to stress. Our sense of humor gives us the ability to find delight, experience joy, and to release tension.

Humor can have a direct link to the spirit or soul. The spirit is the very essence of who we are in the form of finer matter or pure energy.[32] This energy is referred to as "Chi" in the Chinese tradition, as "Ki" in the Japanese tradition. It can be visioned using Kirilian photography, or felt during the application of healing touch. Spirit can be influenced by the feelings of joy, hope and love. The experience of laughter momentarily banishes feelings of anger and fear and provides moments of feeling carefree, lighthearted, and hopeful.

Norman Cousins first called the attention of the medical community to the potential therapeutic effects of humor and laughter in 1979 when he described his utilization of laughter during his treatment for ankylosing spondylitis. Believing that negative emotions had a negative impact on his health, he theorized that the

---

[31] See the chapter: Fear.
[32] See the chapters Before Life/After Death and Angels, Guides and Guidance.

opposite was also true, that positive emotions would have a positive effect. He believed the experience of laughter could open him to feelings of joy, hope, confidence and love.

Cousins, although one of the best known proponents of using positive emotions to improve health, was certainly not the first to assert such a relationship. As early as the 1300's, Henri de Mondeville, professor of surgery wrote:

> **"Let the surgeon take care to regulate the whole regimen of the patient's life for joy and happiness, allowing his relatives and special friends to cheer him, and by having someone tell him jokes."**

The difference is that we now have scientific studies of that relationship. Cousins spent the last 12 years of his life at UCLA Medical School in the Department of Behavioral Medicine exploring the scientific proof of his belief. He established the Humor Research Task Force which coordinated and supported world-wide clinical research on humor.

Stress has been shown to create unhealthy physiological changes. The connection between stress and high blood pressure, muscle tension, immunosuppression and many other changes has been known for years. We now have proof that laughter creates the opposite effects. It appears to be the perfect antidote for stress.

Berk, at Loma Linda University School of Medicine's Dept. of Clinical Immunology, has produced carefully controlled studies showing that the experience of laughter lowers serum cortisol levels, increases the amount of activated T lymphocytes, increases the number and activity of natural killer cells, and increases the number of T cells that have helper/suppresser receptors. In short, laughter stimulates the immune system, off-setting the immunosuppressive effects of stress.

Psychoneuroimmunology defines the communication links and relationships between our emotional experience and our immune response as mediated by the neurological system.

Research has shown that stress, anxiety and depression not only increase levels of immunosuppressive cortisol, they also depress natural killer cell activity, decrease and depress helper T cells. Natural killer cells protect us from cancer and T cells protect us from infections.

Our first-line defense against the entry of infectious organisms through the respiratory tract is salivary immunoglobulin A. Research has clearly demonstrated that salivary immunoglobulin A response level was lower on days of negative mood and higher on days with positive mood. Two groups of researchers found subjects showed an increased concentration of salivary IgA after viewing a humorous video

All this research, done in the last ten years, helps us understand the mind-body connections. The emotions and moods we experience directly effect our immune system. A sense of humor allows us to perceive and appreciate the incongruities of life and provides moments of joy and delight. These positive emotions can create neurochemical changes that will buffer the immunosuppressive effects of stress.

Laughter can provide a cathartic release, a purifying of emotions and release of emotional tension. Laughter, crying, raging and trembling are all cathartic activities which can unblock energy flow.

Humor's Effect on the Mind
In his book, *Stress without Distress*, Selye clarified that a person's interpretation of stress is not dependent solely on an external event, but also depends upon their perception of the event and the meaning they give it—how you look at a situation determines if you will respond to it as threatening or challenging.[33]

Because different people respond differently to the same situations, some people seem to cope with stress better than others. Sociologist Suzanne Kobassa has defined three "hardiness factors" which can increase a person's resilience to stress and

---

[33] See the chapter: Attitude.

prevent burnout: **commitment, control, and challenge**. If you have a strong commitment to yourself and your work, if you believe that you are in control of the choices in your life (internal locus of control), and if you see change as challenging rather than threatening; then you are more likely to cope successfully with stress.

In this context, humor can be an empowerment tool. Humor gives us a different perspective on our problems and, with an attitude of detachment, we feel a sense of self-protection and control in our environment.

> ***"If you can laugh at it, you can survive it."***
> Bill Cosby

Humor and Locus of Control

Patty Wooten's research has shown that if one is encouraged and guided to use humor, they can gain a sense of control in their life.[34] Use of humor represents what Kobassa calls cognitive control. We cannot control events in our external world but we have the ability to control how we view these events and the emotional response we choose to have to them. While no one really knows how humor creates all these positive results we do know that humor perception seems to balance the brain. It involves the whole brain and serves to integrate and balance activity in both hemispheres.

Derks, at the College of William and Mary in Williamsburg, studied brain activity after hearing a joke. During the setup to the joke, the cortex's left hemisphere began its analytical function of processing words received by the auditory center. Shortly afterward, most of the brain activity moved to the frontal lobe which is the center of emotionality. Moments later, the right hemisphere's synthesis capabilities joined with the left's processing to find the pattern—to 'get the joke'. A few

---

[34] Patty Wooten's presented her research in 1990 at the 8th International Conference on Humor in England.

milliseconds later, before the subject had enough time to laugh, the increased brain wave activity spread to the sensory processing areas of the brain, the occipital lobe. The increased fluctuations in delta waves reached a crescendo of activity and crested as the brain 'got' the joke and the external expression of laughter began activating the motor control areas of the brain producing speech from the speech center and muscular movement. Humor pulls the various parts of the brain together rather than activating a component in only one area.

Here is a story Patty Wooten sent for this chapter, it is from her book, *Compassionate Laughter*, Jest for Your Health CommuneAKey Publishing, Salt Lake City, 1996 pg. 8-9.

HOW TO FIND HUMOR

To discover the comic potential in a situation, first see the situation, then recognize it, and then accept it. Gene Perret, in his book, *How to Write and Sell Your Sense of Humor*, suggests that first, you observe the problem or situation carefully. Notice the details. Next, recognize the absurdity or irony present. Ask yourself, who is here? What's going on? Are there power struggles? What are the emotions being experienced? Finally, accept the situation without attempting to control or change it.

I'm reminded of my friend, Frank. He was frequently 10-20 minutes late for work each day. It was difficult for him to arrive at 9 AM because he was a single father with a disabled child. By the time he got his child to school and then drove across town to work, he was often a few minutes late. This didn't seem like a problem, because he worked extra during his lunch hour to make up the time. However, Frank's boss was very controlling and insisted that all employees arrive promptly. One day, the boss chastised Frank in front of his co-workers and announced that if he were ever late again, he would be fired. Frank was embarrassed but vowed to get an earlier start the next day and prevent any tardiness.

Unfortunately, despite of his sincere efforts, he was delayed by a traffic jam and walked into the office at 9:15 AM. His boss stood scowling in the middle of the office and his co-workers anxiously awaited the confrontation. Frank put down his briefcase, walked up to his boss, offered to shake hands and announced, "Hello sir, my name is Frank Jones. I'd like to apply for the position that became available about fifteen minutes ago." After a tense moment, the boss, trying hard to contain a smile, replied, "Just get to work, Frank."

Of course, Frank could have handled the situation in any number of serious ways. But, because he was able to see, recognize and accept the situation, he could create a humorous response to the problem. Frank could see that he was caught, and that there was no way to sneak in unnoticed. He recognized that the boss was not about to lose face by accepting an excuse in front of his co-workers. And finally, Frank accepted that his job was gone, so he had nothing to lose by asking to be his own replacement!

Learning to Laugh

How does one go about laughing? How can one get that humor perspective which can so effect your spirit, mind, and body? How do you learn to access the lighter side of yourself?

Laughing at yourself is not always easy, it is an attitude that is developed. Stay in touch with your "inner clown", that playful, childlike nature that we all have but perhaps fail to acknowledge. Watch children when they play, notice how often they laugh.

Humor and laughter can be effective self-care tools to cope with stress. They can improve the function of the body, the mind, and the spirit. An ability to laugh at our situation or problem gives us hope, serenity and peace. We are less likely to succumb to feelings of depression and helplessness if we are able to laugh at what is troubling us. Humor gives us a sense of perspective on our problems. Laughter provides an opportunity for the release of uncomfortable emotions which, if held inside, may create biochemical changes that are harmful to the body. People can increase their beneficial laughter by adding exposure to humorous material. Humor resources are plentiful. Laughter training exists. We can become our own best medicine.

Jest for the Health of It Services:

Presentations about humor and laughter for health professionals.

Consultation for creating humor programs and laughter libraries.

Patty Wooten, P.O. Box 4040, Davis CA 95617 phone: 916-758-3826

fax: 916-753-7638 or E-Mail to: jestpatty@mother.com

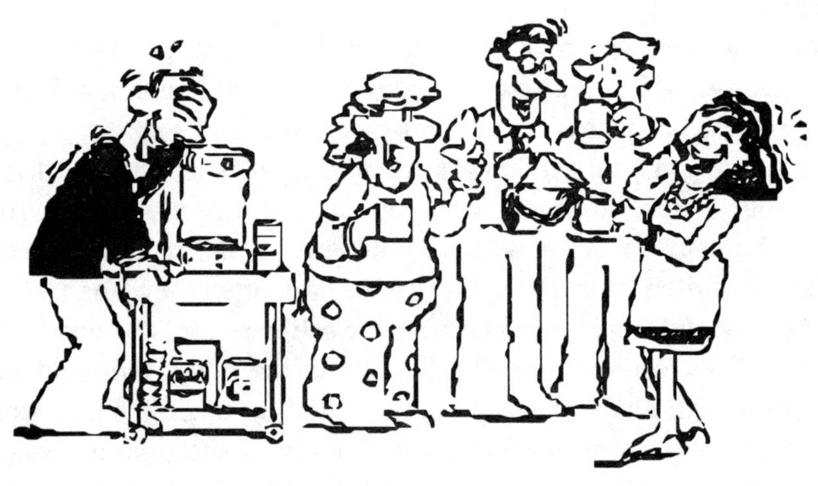

The Twelve Affirmations of Positive Humor
by Christian Hagaseth III, MD
used with permission

1) I am determined to use my humor for positive, playful, uplifting, healing and loving purposes.

2) I will take myself lightly while I take my work in life seriously.

3) I will not seek to be offended by other's attempts at humor. When in doubt, I will see others as meaning well.

4) I will express my humor physically, using my whole face and (when so moved) with my entire body.

5) I refuse to use my humor to camouflage hostility or prejudice.

6) I understand that the gift of laughter is a treasured gift, so I will laugh generously at other's attempts to be humorous.

7) All teasing and ethnic humor will be by mutual consent and will go both ways or I will not engage in such humor.

8) I will respect the forbidden subject topics of my listeners. I will avoid giving offense with my humor.

9) If I offend another by my use of humor, I will make amends.

10) I will be eternally vigilant for the jokes and absurdities of the universe, and I will share my observations with my companions in life.

11) In the midst of adversity, I will continue to use my humor to cope, to survive, to heal, to grow, and to pass on loving-kindness.

12) On the day of my death I will look back and know that I laughed lovingly, fully and well.

HAPPINESS

*"The paradox of achieving personal peace and happiness is
that what we are looking for is already within us.
But, in giving it away we experience it
most powerfully for ourselves."*
—John Marks Templeton

Happiness comes from within, not from without. Choose to be happy by thinking happy thoughts, it is challenging to do this all the time. Happiness takes practice, strength, courage and especially persistence. In any situation in life, there is something good about it. Make it a habit to always look for the good. Happiness is not always having what you want but wanting what you have.

Act as if you are happy and soon you will be. William James said, "Action seems to follow feeling, but really action and feeling go together; and by regulating the action, which is under direct control of the will, we can indirectly regulate feeling, which is not."

Thus the sovereign voluntary path to cheerfulness, if our cheerfulness be lost, is to sit up cheerfully and to **act and speak as if cheerfulness were already there...**"

**"A happy person is not a person in
a certain set of circumstances,
but rather a person with
a certain set of attitudes."**
—Hugh Downs

Two people with the same financial status, family situation and health may be totally different in their levels of happiness. Perception is the key to happiness, I have seen homeless people, disabled people and migrant farm workers who are much happier than doctors, lawyers and CEOs. Shakespeare said, "There is nothing either good or bad, but thinking makes it so." As Abraham

Lincoln once said, "Most folks are about as happy as they make up their minds to be."

"The secret of happiness is not in doing what one likes, but in liking what one does. "—James M. Barrie

Avoid the negative in life, instead of watching the evening news, rent *The Sound of Music* and feed on the happy thoughts.

♥ *I will look for the good in everything ♥ that happens in my life.*

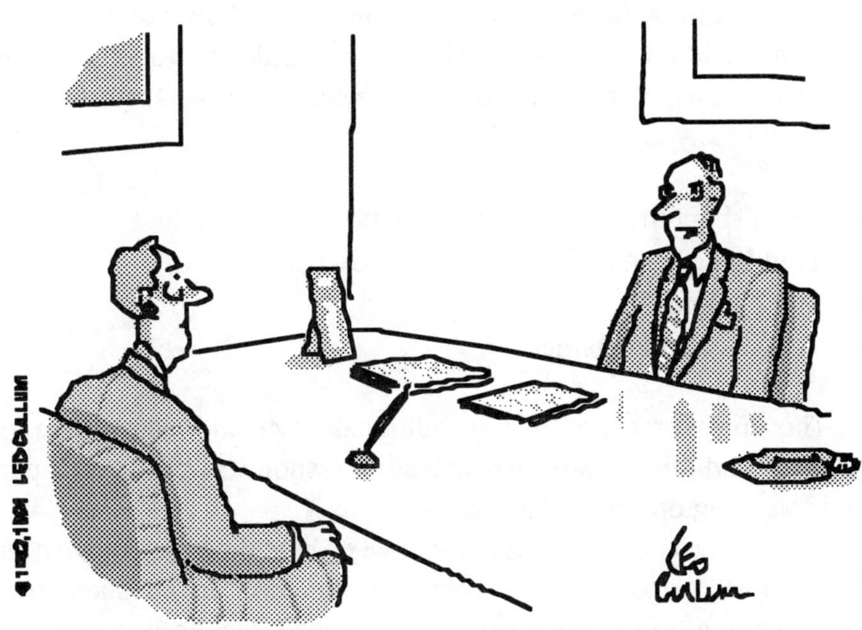

"It's come to my attention that you have a life outside the office."

ANGER

"Everything that irritates us about others can lead us to an understanding of ourselves."
—Carl Jung

Anger can be manifest in our lives in two forms, guilt or resentment. Guilt is anger directed at ourselves for what we did or failed to do (I am bad). Resentment is anger directed at others for what they did or failed to do (They are bad). Guilt can eat us up from the inside out, resentment from the outside in. Not all anger is unhealthy. Anger in either form is a wake up call. Time to look within. Do any of the following fit ?:

- Am I shoulding on myself or others?
- Do I have expectations that are unreal?
- Am I judging?
- Am I assigning blame?

The cure for anger is unconditional love and acceptance of yourself and others. It is also accepting responsibility for your part and forgiving others for their parts.

Anger blocks us from receiving love right at the moment we need it the most. Anger tends to isolate us, we push loved ones away when they are just what we need to speed the healing process. When we are angry we need someone to empathize. Our best Source of empathy is God, then maybe a close friend.

Anger is the master teacher of acceptance, forgiveness and personal responsibility.

FEAR

"Do the thing you fear and death of fear is certain."
—Ralph Waldo Emerson

It has been said that there are only two primary emotions, fear and love. All other emotions are variations of these.

Two of the most important principles in life are:

1. There are no wrong feelings.

2. I cannot make someone feel nor can someone make me feel.

We are responsible for our own feelings. We should never blame anyone for the way we are feeling. There are people in our lives that we hand our heart strings to and say, "go ahead and pull all you want." We have given them power to make us feel. Look at your life, think of someone who you allow to "make you feel." Ask yourself, "If a total stranger did the same thing, would you feel the same way?"

Eleanor Roosevelt once said, "No one can make you feel inferior without your consent." Eleanor also wrote:

"You gain strength, courage and confidence by every experience in which you really stop to look fear in the face."

When we blame others and don't own and take responsibility for our feelings we give our power away. Feelings arise by our perceptions of events in our lives. The event may be perceived differently by other people. Perceptions are based on our beliefs. As a child our parents lovingly taught us to fear new things to keep us safe from danger. Children don't know the difference between poison and food or between friends and strangers. We may have been frightened by strangers or sampling new things like electric sockets or hot coffee. It is likely that fear has saved our lives many times. While these may be rational fears. The fear of new things, of stepping outside our comfort zone, keeps us from living life to the fullest.

Fear is often **F.E.A.R.**—False Evidence Appearing **Real**—a famous acronym that shows us that fear is often just a phantom, not reality.

Fear is always an emotional response to some past experience. ***Fear is never dear and comes from life's rear.*** A tool to take the power out of fear is to trace it's origin. What past event or events caused me to develop this fear? What is the connection to the present situation? Now armed with this knowledge choose your course of action. Step out with courage and have faith that the best will happen.

> ***"Do not look back in anger, or forward in***
> ***fear, but around in awareness."***
> —*James Thurber*

Catastrophising is another aspect of unhealthy fear. This is expecting the worst to happen. Catastrophising is when it goes beyond reality, e.g... "It's going to be awful and terrible and then I'll die." Expectation is a powerful force which will push events in the direction of your expectation. Healthy fear or respect is to look at whatever it is for what it is, and what realistic danger is there. When I am fearful I ask myself, "What is the worst thing that could happen and can I handle that?" This takes the power out of fear.

Most fears are tied into low self-esteem. The fear of rejection, failure or conflict are all blows to your self-esteem. Developing a strong sense of self-worth will protect against these fears. The most common fear is **the fear of abandonment**. A sense of autonomy eliminates this fear. We need to be OK alone and not need someone else in our lives to be complete. Remember, fear is simply a messenger that says stop, look, listen and learn. So, acknowledge your fear and examine it, then step out with courage. Begin the adventure.

♥ ***I will look at my fears realistically and take responsibility.*** ♥

THE COMFORT ZONE

**"A COWARD DIES A HUNDRED DEATHS,
A BRAVE MAN ONLY ONCE."**
—Judge Harry Stone

This is the area in life of familiar people, places, things and activities. If we are not expanding our comfort zone and embracing the new, then this zone is shrinking, trapping us inside.

**"Man cannot discover new oceans until he has the
courage to lose sight of the shore."**
—Anonymous

**"If the primary mission of a captain were
to preserve his ship, he would never leave port."**
—Thomas Aquinas

To live life fully we must have the courage to face the fear of breaking out of our comfort zone. Many people live in a comfort zone. They may live in the same small apartment for years, they only venture out when necessary for the same food they always eat and only listen to the music they are familiar with. Their lives are very predictable. Is this living? Are they fulfilling the measure of their creation and purpose in life? Do they contribute to the world? Do their lives matter?

"Life is either a daring adventure or nothing.
Security does not exist in nature, nor do the
children of men as a whole experience it. Avoiding
danger is no safer in the long run than exposure."
—Helen Keller

In his book *The Road Less Traveled*, psychiatrist Scott Peck observed, "In the struggle to help my patients grow, I found that my chief enemy was invariably their laziness." He noted that people are afraid of change, they are reluctant to "extend to new areas of thought, responsibility and maturation." This fear of stepping out of their comfort zone limits their lives.

> ***"If nothing is ventured, nothing is gained."***
> —Sir John Heywood

Live your lives fully, face your fears and expand your comfort zone. If you feel resistance to action or new ideas, look at it carefully. Is it fear only? Then face your fears and go against the resistance. Expanding your comfort zone will keep you young in body, mind and spirit.

> ***"People are always blaming circumstances for
> what they are. I do not believe in
> circumstances.
> The people who get on in this world are the
> people who get up and look for the
> circumstances they want,
> and if they cannot find them make them."***
> —George Bernard Shaw

RELATIONSHIPS

True love is unconditional, it is not based on performance.

We have everything **now** that we need to be complete. A misconception is—that we need something from another person, and we will love that person when we get it, or hate them if we don't. Many relationships are based on trading conditional love. The motivation to get instead of give leads to conflict and distress. Happiness comes from within, no person, place or thing is responsible for your joy.

Let go of judging, accept people as they are. Don't try to force them into your mold. Remember, control and domination are not love. Love is to let someone go and be. Let go of attachments, nothing and no one truly belong to you.[35] **If you love something, set it free, if it comes back it is yours, if it doesn't come back it wasn't yours to begin with.**

To be lovable is to be loving.

Communication is an essential tool for healthy relationships. Ask for what you need, don't expect your partner to read your mind. Know when to say something and when to practice silence. Listen more; talk less. God gave us a hint when He gave us two ears and one mouth.

John Gray in his book, *Men are from Mars, Women are from Venus,* points out the difference in male vs. female communication. Women expect to be listened to without a man trying to "fix" her or solve her problems. Men need to realize that after she has talked things out and felt that she has been heard, she will be "fixed." Men

---

[35] See the chapter: Detachment.

on the other hand will often not talk until they have either solved the problem or realized they need help, then they will talk. Trying to make the man talk will frustrate the woman and anger the man. Have patience, he will come out of his cave. Don't tell a man what to do or a woman how she should feel.

The most powerful communication skill is empathy. Empathy is actually understanding how someone feels, sympathy is feeling for them eg.: "I feel sorry for you." **Strive to be empathetic not sympathetic.**

I was having dinner one night with two young ladies Kayla, age 9 and Krystle, age 10. They were telling me how they felt sorry for a friend of theirs that was crippled and just now learning to walk with braces. When I explained to them—*it isn't good to feel for other people* and we *let them feel for themselves*, they thought I was mean and cruel. I continued to explain to them that she was probably happy that she could now walk. I told them that *emotionally healthy people don't want pity or sympathy.* Krystle and Kayla found these ideas challenging to understand until they asked their friend if she was happy and if she wanted people to feel sorry for her. The answers they received were great lessons. This inspiring young lady, who recently walked a mile in a local parade twirling a baton, told them she was happy and she didn't want anyone feeling sorry for her.

The Law of Mirroring and Projecting: We tend to see in others and in the world, that which is within ourselves. We often project our characteristics onto others. If we see only the good, we have changed for the better within.

Sometimes we don't like what we see in the mirror. Remember the first time you heard your voice on a tape recorder or saw yourself on videotape. Did you say, "I don't sound like that or look like that?" Were you your own worst critic? The mirror is similar, when we really look, we may not like what we see. We must accept who we are before we can make any changes.[36]

> ***"If you want to make the world a better place,***
> ***take a look at yourself and then make a change. "***
> Michael Jackson's song, *Man in the Mirror*

One example of mirroring is jealousy, if someone is often feeling jealous in a relationship, it is likely that he or she doesn't trust themselves. They are projecting unfaithful behavior onto their mate because they question their own ability to be faithful. The singer Laurel Lee says, "I know I'm not seeing things as they are, I'm seeing things as I am."

In the 7th chapter, verses 1-5 of Matthew, Jesus is concluding the sermon on the mount. He tells us not to judge others because that same judgment will be used for us. He says, however we measure or evaluate others, that is how we will be evaluated. Why do you look at the speck of dust in your brother's eye and pay no attention to the plank in your own eye? How can you say to your brother, "Let me take the speck out of your eye," when all the time there is a plank in your own eye? You hypocrite, first take the plank out of your own eye, and then you will see clearly to remove the speck from your brother's eye.

> ***"Mirrors should reflect a little***
> ***before throwing back images. "***
> —Jean Cocteau

If you are making harsh judgments of other people, whatever advice you would give them is the advice you need for yourself. I am actually writing this book for me, I need every scrap of advice in it. It is my desire for personal growth that inspires me to write,

---

[36] See the chapter: Acceptance.

speak and counsel. Perhaps the reason I enjoy counseling is that it gives me opportunities to learn more about me.

> **"I bid him look into the lives of men as though looking into a mirror, and from others to take an example for himself."**
> —Terence, 190-159 B.C.

My closest friend has a sister that is content to do nothing with her life. She is seventeen and has only finished 9th grade. She had a job in a fast food restaurant, this only lasted a couple months—she is happy to cook and clean for her father. When her sister calls and complains about her life my friend listens and helps her find solutions—unfortunately the sister never follows through. My friend feels intense anger—a red flag of something deep inside herself—mirroring.

> **"When we see men of contrary character, we should turn inward and examine ourselves."**
> —Confucius

My friend and I discussed the source of her anger, it became evident that there had been a similar situation in her life that was being mirrored. Most of her life she had felt trapped. At age seventeen, she became a mother and soon had two daughters, her husband was in the Navy and off on a ship. In another marriage, her husband sabotaged her car to keep her trapped at home. It wasn't until she broke out of the trap, (welfare mother situation) that things began to change. She went back to school and volunteered her time to get work experience. Now, she has a good job as a medical office manager and a strong healthy relationship.

What does this have to do with her sister? It was those memories of being trapped and not knowing how to get free. Her sister has opportunities but does nothing to advance herself. This is the root of her anger.

"A loving person lives in a loving world.
A hostile person lives in a hostile world.
Everyone you meet is your mirror."
—Ken Keyes, *Handbook to Higher Consciousness*

The mirror also has a positive side, the beauty and good we see in others and the world is a reflection of what is beautiful and good in ourselves. Look for the good. Pay attention to the negative, in as much as it may teach you something about yourself.

"We really don't learn anything from our experience.
We only learn from reflecting on our experience."
—Robert Sinclair

LOVE : Love is not caring for people, it is caring about them. M. Scott Peck, M.D. defines love as: "The will to extend one's self for the purpose of nurturing one's own or another's spiritual growth."

The Greeks developed several definitions of love: Eros— romantic love; Storge—family love; Phileo—love of friends; and **Agape—unselfish love.** Agape is the love that Christ taught us, it is unconditional and expects nothing in return.

Agape is magical in that, the more you give
the more you have to give.

PASSION: naturally goes in cycles. The cycle is bonding followed by separation. Alone time is fundamental to passion. Continuous bonding weakens the passion, both partners need to have their own lives. To keep passion alive takes work. Relationships can become boring if everything is always the same.

Use your imagination and create newness and variety in your relationships.

Constantly courting your mate is essential to maintaining a romantic relationship. Women need to feel special and feminine, they want to be romanced they love flowers, candlelight dinners etc. Women and men need touching without sexual motives. Men need to feel masculine and that they make a difference—they need to feel that their mates are happy. Instead of guessing, ask your mate what they want and tell them what you want.

"Happy relationships depend not on finding the right person, but being the right person."
—Eric Butterworth

Tips For Happier Relationships

Appreciate one another! The desire for appreciation is one of the deepest of all human cravings. Use loving words and actions. If you don't, you might wake up one morning and wonder what happened—by then it will be too late. Let he or she know they're still attractive to you. Don't stifle the urge to hold hands, hug or kiss!

Respect each other's opinions, beliefs, ideas and desires. Stop thinking you can force them to change. They'll only resent you for it. Let them do it themselves. Trust that they have their own resources for change. Be patient—it may take awhile!

Grow gracefully with one other. Respect their timing. It is more than likely different than your own! Grant them their birthright of individuality. Only they know what's best for themselves, even if you are sure you do!

Men—cherish and reassure your woman.
Women—trust, admire and accept your man.

* Put yourself and your spouse, family and partner before work. Put your significant other before children. If you don't someone you love may start packing! [37]

* Do not assume anything—stop expecting him or her to be a mind-reader. Ask for what you want in a direct way.

* Take time to air your feelings. Holding them in will only create distance and resentment. Talk it out. You can find the way to work things out.

* Trust each other. If this is difficult for you, seek counseling or professional help. There are many support groups, or talk with a close friend. Without trust, there can be no love.

* Remember in your early days? You were friends—right? If you find yourself being more of a mom or a dad to your loved one, stop before you destroy your love. Do what it takes to re-establish your friendship. You'll have a lot more fun!

Friends laugh and cry together, prop each other up when the chips are down. Friends don't pester or pretend. They can be themselves when they're with one another. True friends respect each other's values, beliefs, feelings and opinions whether or not they agree with them. They are not obsessed with being "right."

* Real friends display gentleness and compassion when their friend is down. They cherish and treasure their friendship above all else. True friends are loyal, devoted and honest. They support you in what you want to do. They wouldn't oppose you without good reason. True friends are kind and listen with open hearts to what's hurting you. They don't flog you with words of blame, judgment and criticism. A real friend will love you unconditionally. So—if

---

[37] Putting your spouse before the children does not mean to allow child abuse.

you want your friend to stay around for awhile, accept him or her "as is."

* Act as equals. Stop competing, comparing and criticizing.

* Create rituals and ceremonies together and with your family. Celebrate birthdays, anniversaries, and holidays in your own unique way. Dream up special occasions!

* Be **flexible** enough to shift gears if the situation calls for it.

* Be his **helpmate**, not his slave. He will respect you much more when you establish that. And, you'll respect yourself. Besides, if you're behaving like the guy's mom, he's not going to feel romantically inclined—if you know what I mean! No one wants to make love with their mom.

* Be one another's lover, friend and confidante. That'll keep the sparks flying!

* Make it safe for your mate to be **vulnerable**, allow yourself be vulnerable

* Spend time together playing, laughing, talking, walking together, anything that creates closeness. Snuggle up, read side by side or do some other activity near each other. Take him or her on a surprise mid-afternoon date, etc. Remember spontaneity!? Take a weekend vacation to somewhere you've never been. You needn't go far. Stay at a local bed and breakfast or in a honeymoon cottage. Bring each other a fair share of joy!

* Write, fax or e-mail each other love notes. If you write notes, put them in unusual places, it adds to the excitement.

* Be spontaneous—surprise each other with little gifts and notes often! Men—do bring flowers, especially wildly colored big fat bouquets—women love them! Women—be the aggressor and show your man that you want and desire him!

* Contemplate one another's admirable qualities. Then write them down and exchange notes.

* Think before you speak—is it true? Is it kind? Is it necessary? If not, let it be left unsaid.

* Have beautiful thoughts, for they may break into words at any moment!

* Validate each other's feelings. Tell him or her that you know they're not imagining things, and that yes, it is real if he or she is experiencing it, whatever it may be.

* Let one another know when a job is well done.

* Have faith in him or her and let them know that you do!

* Allow for individual strengths and differences. Give each other space. Respect one another's need for privacy and solitude.

* And, most important of all, **"The Law Of Allowing."** Allow your loved ones the time and space to do whatever it is they need to do without judging or advising them. It's not always easy to do! However, this is essential for better relationships. If you do nothing else but this, your relationships will improve dramatically.

I will take the time and thought to nourish my relationship.

COMMUNICATION

The rules for being an excellent communicator are quite simple—**listen, be interested and be sincere.** Putting these into practice takes time, effort and commitment. I will personally guarantee, it will be worth it—your whole life will change. You will be more successful in work, as a mate and as a parent.

Listening will solve more problems than any amount of speaking ever could. Listen openly, attentively and empathetically. Really try to understand what the other person is saying. Put yourself in their shoes and understand what they are feeling. It is best to let them talk until they are finished. Then, paraphrase what they've said and ask them if it is right. If you have difficulty empathizing or understanding ask "why" questions.

The easiest way to be a good conversationalist is to ask good questions, showing interest. Larry King, the host of *Larry King Live* is a master of this. He is, the only TV phone-in talk show host. In his book, *How to Talk to Anyone, Anytime, Anywhere—The Secrets of Good Communication* he states that his favorite question is—Why? He says, "It's the greatest question ever asked, and it always will be. And it is certainly the surest way of keeping conversation lively and interesting."

People crave attention, so much so that they will often go to the doctor to get it. I have seen it in my own practice. Give people attention through listening and showing an interest and you will have a friend.

If you want people to **avoid you**, **laugh at you** and **dislike you** follow this formula given by Dale Carnegie:

> *"Never listen to anyone for long. Talk incessantly about yourself. If you have an idea while the other person is talking, don't wait for them to finish—bust right in and interrupt in the middle of a sentence."*

Before speaking, think, especially when dealing with an issue involving your partner or another person. Become aware of your thoughts, feelings and any intuitive insights you might have around the issue. What do you want to convey? What **do** you want?

Ten Rules for Relationship Communication
(For dealing with specific challenging issues)

1. Out of fairness and respect, choose a mutually convenient time and place to discuss **one issue only**. Agree on which issue will be discussed, and on the length of your session.

2. Don't be an **archeologist** by digging up the past, or a **fortune teller** by predicting the future. Stick to the present issue.

3. Beforehand, prepare and calm yourself. Do your favorite meditation or relaxation technique, or simply take 4 very deep breaths and let them out slowly. Perhaps take a walk or do some stretches or some kind of movement to relax your body. If you have time, soak in a hot tub or take a relaxing shower.

4. Maintain relaxed eye contact. Remember to blink and breathe! Check in often to see whether you're relaxed or tense. Tensing, then letting go of your neck and shoulder muscles helps. Making large circles with your shoulders, forward and backwards helps too. Raising and alternately knitting your eyebrows then letting go will relieve scalp and forehead tightness. Opening and closing your mouth helps jaw tension. Use whatever works for you! Maybe you need to change where or how you're sitting. Make whatever adjustments might be necessary, take time out and agree on when to start again.

5. Stay in touch with what you are thinking and feeling.

6. Become clear of your intentions. What do you **want**?

7. With a pleasant tone of voice (no whining!), use "I" statements. This takes it out of the blaming, judging arena. Ask yourself a

few questions: "Do I want to fight?" **"Am I insisting on being right, no matter what?"** "Or, would I rather create an atmosphere of mutual trust, safety and understanding?" "Am I coming from a place of love or fear?" If it is fear and you feel safe, go ahead and talk about your fears—it is OK to be vulnerable. If feeling angry or over-reactive, let the other know and reschedule your time together. Then breathe deeply, take a walk, or whatever it takes to get you calmed down and rational.

8. Ask the other person to repeat back what you have just said. They may have incorrectly heard and/or misinterpreted your communication. This crucial step will give you more clarity and understanding around the issue.

9. Brainstorm for solutions. Open up to creative ideas that may not occur to you normally. Be willing to **compromise**. Agree on at least one step you can take to immediately resolve or at least relieve the tensions around the issue. Give each other a big hug! And **let them know how much you love and appreciate them.**

10. Do not be discouraged if the resolution is incomplete at this time. Reschedule to come back to the issue again, if necessary. Commit to take as long as it takes to be resolved or at least relieved. At the end of your "session" you will feel empowered knowing you have taken vital steps toward having what you want.

HOW TO WIN FRIENDS & INFLUENCE PEOPLE

Over thirty years ago, Dale Carnegie wrote *How to Win Friends & Influence People*, it has since sold over 15,000,000 copies. I believe it should be required reading for anyone that wants to be happy and successful.

These principles have been taught over and over again by hundreds of successful writers and lecturers. Use them well and it will change your life.

Never criticize, condemn or complain—ask yourself how you feel about people that don't follow this principle. Negative thinking is the hallmark of an unhappy person. This negative thinking tends to attract more negative into that person's life as well as to drive away the positive.

Be appreciative—when a person is sincerely appreciative of another person, that person will want to do more for them. They will also tend to like that person. Dale Carnegie kept this old saying on his mirror:

"I shall pass this way but once; any good, therefore, that I can do or any kindness that I can show to any human being, let me do it now. Let me not defer nor neglect it, for I shall not pass this way again."
—William Penn

Help others to get what they want, while getting what you want. An old Hindu proverb says: Help thy brother's boat across, and lo—Thy own has reached the shore. People are generally not interested in what you want, they are interested in what they want. If you can create win/win situations in giving and getting, you will get what you want. Sometimes what you want comes in conflict with someone else's want. You **can** compromise and create a win/win solution. The better you understand the other person the easier this will be. Henry Ford elicited this marvelous advice in relationships:

> *"If there is any one secret to success, it lies in the ability to get the other person's point of view and see things from that person's angle as well as your own."*

Be genuinely interested in other people—Dale Carnegie said, "You can make more friends in two months by becoming interested in other people than you can in two years trying to get them interested in you." Alfred Adler a famous psychiatrist said, "It is the individual who is not interested in his fellow men who has the greatest difficulties in life and provides the greatest injury to others. It is from among such individuals that all human failures spring."

Smile—Actions speak louder than words, a smile says—I like you. I feel happy when you are here. Smiling puts people at ease and people who smile are much more effective leaders, teachers and parents. Employers, myself included, would rather hire a person with no schooling and a pleasant smile than a Ph.D. with a somber face.

Remember the person—I can remember a doctor from my early training as a resident. When I followed him in his office he could remember all of his patients, not just their names, but something about them. I marveled that this man had such a great memory. I asked him how he did it, he said, "I don't have any better memory than you, I just take notes." He wrote a little note in each patient's chart about them. Remembering names doesn't come easy to most people, it takes caring and effort.

"Remember that a person's name is to that person the sweetest and most important sound in any language."
—Dale Carnegie

**"Talk to people about themselves
and they will listen for hours."**
—Disraeli

Listen and encourage others to talk about themselves and their interests—people want respect, appreciation and to know that they matter. If you can make someone feel important to you they will be open and willing to help and serve you. All the great prophets taught this and Jesus summed it up nicely:

*"Do unto others as you would have
others do unto you."*

Be courteous—remember please and thank you. If you show appreciation for whatever is done for you then it will likely be repeated.

Create Win/Win situations—because there are no win/lose or lose/win situations in personal and most business relations; there are only win/win or lose/lose situations. One person may believe they have won a conflict but damage occurs to the relationship whenever there is a loser. Arguments and confrontation usually produce anger, hurt and resentment. The "winner" of an argument may feel good about his triumph but will the loser? No, he will resent his "enemy."

*"If you argue and rankle and contradict,
you may achieve a victory sometimes; but it
will be an empty victory because you will
never get your opponent's good will"*
—Benjamin Franklin

How many friendships, relationships and businesses have been destroyed by arguments and false pride? Disagreement creates defensiveness in both people—winning becomes their only goal. There will be no empathy, no genuine listening and certainly no openness to the others ideas.

> ***"A man convinced against his will***
> ***is of the same opinion still."***
> Dale Carnegie

To win someone to your way of thinking, agree with him and patiently listen. Wait until he has finished his point, tell him how you agree with him. Next, present your thoughts. By doing this, two things will happen. First, more than half the time you will learn something that may change **your** mind. Second, the other person will be more receptive to your ideas.

Remember the saying, two heads are better than one? This is true because two people will have two different ideas about the same thing. Disagreements are good, they force us to think, examine our ideas and make better choices.

For eight years I was the only foot specialist for the Southern Oregon coast. I now have my associate, Dr. William Bennett working with me. Dr. Bennett brings his own unique experiences to the practice. When we see a patient together we may have different treatment plans. We discuss the patient's problem and all the options for treatment. By this process, we learn how to serve our patients better. If either us was arrogant or prideful, we would be damned from this type of learning.

A true sign of an advanced spiritual being
is their humble, teachable and loving nature.

Without these qualities we become defensive when questioned.

Children can give parents opportunities to learn patience. Someone once said, "If you pray for patience, God will send you children." I have five biological children and two others that I am dad to. My seventeen year old son, Jared has taught me the most about arguing. It is natural for teenagers to question authority. Some parents argue, nag, lecture and complain, and get nowhere. Listening, empathizing and helping youngsters get what they need, will get us what we want—peace, serenity and joy. Teens, children, and adults want to be understood, respected and loved unconditionally. There is no perfect parent.

If your children—or any human
can feel understood, respected and loved
unconditionally then, you are doing a great job.

Making an enemy—one of the surest ways to show disrespect and to make an enemy is to tell someone they are wrong. When you call them a liar, you strike down their pride, self-esteem and intelligence. Instead of telling somebody they are wrong ask them questions that will lead them to the truth. It is always best to get people to agree with you. Make people your friends not your opponents.

When you have a disagreement, admit you might be wrong, this takes them off the defensive. Now, you can both openly examine the facts and have a healthy and productive discussion. Remain humble, teachable and kindhearted.

Be responsible—responsibility (response-ability) is the hallmark of a mature person. When you are wrong or make a mistake, admit it quickly and emphatically. The greatest qualities in employees are good people skills, a pleasant disposition and a great sense of responsibility. The best employee I ever had took responsibility not only for her mistakes but for the others she managed. She went even farther to confess a mistake that she could have easily covered up. I have much more respect for these qualities than for someone that never admits to making mistakes.

Think about it—how could anyone be angry with someone that comes to you and humbly admits a mistake and takes full responsibility for it.

Influence—if you want to help someone's performance, a child, spouse or business associate, give them praise. People crave praise and appreciation, the average person gets too little. Most of us will double our efforts and go out of our way for someone who gives us **sincere praise and honest appreciation.** There is a law I learned in psychology and in books about raising children. That law is—self fulfilling prophecy. We become whatever we believe we are. We can change these beliefs.[38] This law states that each of us rise to our own expectations. Those expectations come from deep within us. They are created by our experiences in life, or our perception of those experiences. We choose how we perceive all life events. Some of us choose to be victims, possessing no real power of our own. Others, choose to see adverse events as challenges that will make us strong.

Often, the most influence we experience is what others think about us. Adults choose who to give this power to. As children, the power is in the hands of parents, educators and friends. Children are greatly influenced by what they perceive others think about them. If they are labeled dumb, irresponsible and immature they are likely to be that. If told they are intelligent, capable and responsible they will rise to those expectations. Regarding undesirable behavior—"Praise the child, condemn the behavior." This also works with mates. When we communicate in our words and actions that they are beautiful, sexy and desired, they will be. In business—show sincere praise and honest appreciation for others. The result will be better productivity, loyalty and a pleasant workplace.

Your power to influence is proportional to your ability to give sincere praise and honest appreciation.

---

[38] see the chapter: on Visualization

BELIEF, THE POWER OF POSITIVE THINKING

"As a man thinketh, so shall he be"

Believe in yourself or no one else will. Throughout this book I have talked about belief and positive thinking. Norman Vincent Peale in his book, *The Power of Positive Thinking,* gave ten easy rules for overcoming inadequacy attitudes and learning to practice faith. Here are ten rules I have written as inspired by Dr. Peale:

1. Visualize yourself as you want to be. Clearly define this picture and carve it into stone in your mind. Don't let it slip or become—maybe or someday. Visualize it as, now I am.

2. As doubts and fears slip into your mind, cancel them and replace them with this positive visualization of your future self.

3. When obstacles appear, be grateful for the challenge. Have courage and faith, don't let your fears stop you. In your mind, minimize these obstacles and see yourself winning and overcoming them.

4. Study other people that you admire. Follow their success formulas as they fit into your personality. Remember, they are no better than you. The only difference is they had a purpose—a plan and a road map for getting there. You now have the same road map and plan, learn from their mistakes, make your own and don't repeat theirs.

5. Repeat the affirmations in the affirmation chapter each morning and evening. Dr. Peale recommends saying these affirmations out loud ten times a day:

📖 "If God be for us who can be against us?" (Romans 8:31)

📖 "I can do all things through Christ which strengtheneth me." (Phillippians 4:13)

📖 "the kingdom of God is within me" (Luke 17:21)

6. Have a healthy concept of God, and visualize Him being with you. Feel His presence and thank Him for being there. If you don't feel comfortable with the concept of God or are unsure read the chapters: Before Birth/After Death and Angels, Guides and Guidance.
7. When you pray, don't say things such as please help me or please be with me—say thank you for helping me, thank you for being here.
8. Find a good counselor. Most people need a coach—a spiritual counselor to help them understand their behavior and feelings. Find the roots of any inferiority and self doubt feelings. Learn to erase this programming from your mind and replace it with positive programming. **Self knowledge is personal power.**
9. Beware of any church, counselor or other that produce negative thinking.
10. Make a true estimate of your own ability, then raise it 10 percent. Do it! Allow no thoughts of failure like—I'll try. **Try** leaves you open to failure.

Belief is the most powerful force in the universe

"Go thy way, and as thou hast believed
so shall it be done unto him."
Jesus

DETACHMENT

Our greatest block to happiness and inner peace is over our attachments, dependency or codependency to people, places and things. Letting go of the "Things of the world" will truly make us free and paradoxically allow us to enjoy these people, places and things more fully.

Possessions can complicate our lives. They can cause us to focus more on acquisition and accumulation than on love and service to humanity. Jesus taught us that where our treasures are, that is where our heart is.

"Lay not up for yourselves treasures upon earth, where moth and rust doth corrupt, and where thieves break through and steal: But lay up for yourselves treasures in heaven, where neither moth nor rust corrupt, and where thieves do not break through nor steal : For where your treasure is, there will your heart be also."
(Matthew 6:19-21)

Many of us believe money and "things" will make us happy. Often, the contrary is true. Riches can isolate us and lead to loneliness. Without mentioning any names, look at the rich and famous. Has fame and fortune brought them happiness? I believe there are more happy poor than happy rich. I am not saying that possessions or money are evil, it is our attachment to it that binds us. Once, I lived in the world of "I'll be happy when", well, when came, I had everything I wanted and I still wasn't happy. It wasn't until everything was stripped away that I began to grow spiritually. This reminds me of what Jesus once said, "It is easier for a camel to pass through the eye of a needle than for a rich man to enter the kingdom of Heaven." The eye of a needle was a very small geologic formation, not an actual needle. The interesting paradox is—once you grow spiritually you often attract wealth.

"The love of money is the root of all evil."
(1 Tim 6:10)

Money is not evil, it is the love of it. Money is only a tool, it can be used to do good or bad depending on the person using it.

Attachments to the physical world will bind us to that world. Almost all pain and sorrow has its roots in attachment. Once we let go we can soar spiritually.

The most difficult detachment (for me anyway) is detaching from loved ones. Detachment doesn't mean not caring, it means caring enough to let your loved one follow their own path while loving them unconditionally.[39] If you feel the need to own and control another this is attachment. Also, needing someone else in your life to feel complete is attachment. Let go of your expectations of others and the closer and more loving you will become. Another great binding attachment is to the past or to the familiar. These attachments prevent change and growth.[40]

Releasing the past means not blaming anyone, including ourselves. It means holding no grievances and totally accepting everyone as is, no exceptions.

Let Go and Let God

---

[39] See the chapter: Relationships.
[40] See the chapters: Change and Comfort Zone.

PRAYER

"Doctors don't know everything really. They understand matter, not spirit. And you and I live in the spirit."
—William Saroyan

There are several doctors who believe in the power of prayer, in fact, many have written books about it. Larry Dossey, M.D. wrote the book *Healing Words* about the power of prayer and the practice of medicine. Dr. Dossey examined hundreds of scientific studies on prayer, many of these were double blind studies. Double blind studies were done with one group being prayed for and another not. Neither doctors, nurses nor patients knew which group they were in. He found that prayer strongly influenced healing and other physiological processes in the body. These effects occurred whether or not the patient knew about the prayer or if the people praying knew the patient. These phenomenal effects were not just limited to humans, they were also demonstrated in plants, animals, bacteria, fungi, seeds and more. Distance was not a factor, the effects could be invoked locally or at a distance. Prayer was so powerful that an object could be placed in a lead lined room that shielded it from all known forms of electromagnetic energy, the effect still got through.

Dr. Dossey found that the most effective prayer was to pray for the best outcome and not prayers for specific outcomes.

Based on my own research and experiences I give you this guide to prayer and one example of my own prayer:

How to pray:

Express gratitude for all that you have and in advance for all you expect to receive **as if you have already received it.**

Always be open for guidance to your highest path. Seek God's will not your own. We may think we know what is best for us or what will make us happy eg. "I'll be happy when." Our true path to happiness comes in fulfilling our purpose—our destiny.

The essence of prayer is not what is said, but in the connecting with your higher power. This connection is best established through regular prayer followed by solitude and meditation. As I have said before, God gave us two ears and only one mouth, perhaps this is a subtle hint that we should spend more time listening and less time talking.

Brian's Prayer

I am grateful for my trials & tribulations for they have shaped my character and stimulated my spiritual growth. I am becoming more courageous. I am thankful for my many mistakes for they have taught me so much. I am responsible for everything I have created in my life. I blame no person, place or thing for my situation in life. I greatly appreciate the guidance you have always given me to my highest path. My vision is becoming clear.

Thank you for always being by my side and lighting my way through all my fears, frustrations and darkness. My faith gives me hope for I know that everything that happens in my life is for my highest good. I let go of worry and face my challenges. I am becoming more one with God and the universe.

Your unconditional love warms my heart. I let go of judging and show compassion & empathy to all my brothers & sisters.

I am forgiven for all my imperfections. I forgive everyone in my life for in forgiveness I find serenity and peace of mind.

I send my love and light to anyone who may have done something to hurt or offend me.

I am a channel of your love it is the purpose of my life to give love.

MEDITATION

*A brief introduction in how to meditate
and ways to improve meditation.*

The primary purposes of meditation are to reconnect with God, develop cosmic consciousness, and to experience self-realization.

Meditation is a technique of using a focus to help quiet the mind—the incessant stream of images, thoughts which seem to be in our heads. Physical and emotional benefits are:

1. *Healing of the body.*
2. *Stress reduced.*
3. *The Inner Voice felt and heard.*
4. *Enlightenment.*
5. *Understanding your life's purpose and path.*

The basis of meditation is choosing something to focus on—*a thought, a sound, an object, a visualization, the breath, or whatever*—and keep your awareness on that point. **Whenever the mind wanders off your focus, refocus. Eventually, by this process of focusing and refocusing on one point;**

1. **The internal noise is lessened.**
2. **Your head is quieter.**
3. **Your energy higher.**

Deeper levels of meditation begin after the initial noise and distracting thoughts have been cleared away. Usually, **periods of quiet**—when it's easy to focus—**alternate** with periods of random thinking. As you **continue to meditate,** *times of easier focus, greater clarity, inner quiet lengthens.* **These times of quiet**

are the first goals of meditation. There is *no limit to the depth and energy that can be found in meditation.*

Any meditation should be continued until a quiet place is reached. *Don't stop when it's difficult to concentrate, in the midst of alot of thoughts.* Stop when you are quiet. **These periods of noise and quiet will alternate as your meditation breaks through layers of thought and tensions of the day.** So stop whenever a more stable place is reached. *You don't have to reach Nirvana to have a great meditation.*

Four easy ways to meditate

1. **Mantras—An easy, common mantra is *OM*,** pronounced with a long oooh and a short mm sound. Dr. Herbert Benson in his excellent book *The Relaxation Response*, recommends using the number one.
2. **Breath focus—**You can choose to **watch your breath, focusing on the inhale and the exhale.** Just pay attention to the inhale and the exhale and *keep your eyes relaxed and open, gazing at the floor or wall a few feet in front of you.*
3. **Focal point—**You can pick a point on a blank wall, a mandala[41] or any object a foot or so in front of you. Or *gaze at a candle flame.*
4. **Meditations on the third eye—**the point between the eyes and about an inch above them in the middle of the forehead—or **the crown chakra,**[42] the top of the head—*are examples of internally focused meditations.* Choose a method that appeals to you. *Find the technique which seems to give you the most energy. Find the right key to your inner lock.*

Meditation allows us to move out of everyday awareness into *higher states of mind and being.* To enter the meditative state with

---

[41] An American Indian tool for meditation.
[42] See the chapter: Chakras.

the breath technique—breathe slowly and fully, following the breath as it enters the nostrils and moves through the body. Concentrate on relaxing more deeply with each breath to quiet the body, mind, emotions, allowing the self to expand into higher awareness. Some people use a mantra, some a mandala, some use a certain inner symbol or vision and some count. The point is to be able to focus awareness into a quiet, peaceful place beyond the intellectual inner dialogue of everyday concerns, worries, doubts and fears. Guided group meditations or tapes are a good places to learn this practice.

We use this time of meditation to move out of ordinary awareness and into a peaceful state of being. We should meditate with an intention of experiencing some part of our higher inner landscape, a more spiritual view of our present situations and possible futures. Eventually, we learn how to go into this state of peace and detachment from the everyday to ask questions of our higher selves and guidance about handling life situations, our jobs, our relationships, our bad habits in a newer and better way.

Quieting the mind, stopping the inner dialogue of the intellect, takes some practice. We are all too used to and dependent upon verbal communication. We are habituated to environmental noise: TV's, radios, audio inputs, computers, telephones, household sounds, the voices, needs and wants of our families, friends, neighbors and business associates. We are used to being pulled off-center and out of inner focus into forgetfulness. Recorded guided meditations, quiet music, a waterfall or some combination of light, sound and aromatherapy scents are helpful to distract us from this on-going, intrusive cacophony of outer concerns and lower mental dialogue. When being quiet becomes a habit, we are open to hear our higher minds and guidance speak to and through us.

Regardless of how you meditate, there are ways to improve meditation. Sitting in a straight back chair with your *back and* *neck straight will make the energy flow more easily through your spine.* Find a fairly comfortable position to sit in.

Start your meditation with your energy as high as possible. *It's nice to have showered first. Feel awake.* **The higher your energy is, the more awake and alert you feel, then the easier it will be to focus and meditate.** *It's best to meditate after eating a light meal, preferably fruit.* If you are hungry it will be difficult to focus and a large meal especially fats and/or carbohydrates will make you sleepy.

Choose a quiet time of day, if you can. Ear plugs are wonderful even if you are repeating a mantra. **Meditation is all about breaking through the everyday world of tension and thoughts to create greater inner peace, calm, insight, and enlightenment;** *find the method or methods which suit you best.*

Choose a time frame to meditate for at least 15 or 20 minutes. My favorite times are first thing in the morning after drinking fresh squeezed fruit juice, lunch time and right before I retire at night. Don't be too rigid in your practice; sometimes you may realize more and feel better by doing something totally different such as listening to peaceful calming music or going for a walk on the beach or in a safe park. Remember that **repetition is the key to mastery.** *Be consistent and committed.*. It takes about *21 consecutive days* of practicing something to **establish a new habit.**

The National Institutes of Health N.I.H. has recently reported that **meditation is the most effective method** for treating the chronic pain of the lower back, arthritis and headaches.

Another of Technique of Meditation

- Sit at ease in any posture.

- Close your eyes and gaze straight ahead in a relaxed and alert manner. Watch whatever space you perceive after closing your eyes.
- Silently repeat the words Amaram Hum Madhuram Hum, which means "I am immortal, I am blissful," as if the words are coming from the space towards your eyes. Put your attention on the space or gap between Amaram Hum and Madhuram Hum. This space is the source or ocean out of which all waves of existence and consciousness arise.
- If any thoughts, feelings, emotions, or visions appear, or if any sounds are heard, just watch these waves without feeling interrupted or disturbed; every wave is a part of your meditation experience. And if no experiences arise, remain alert; this pure space is the ocean of consciousness, without any ripple on its surface.
- Remain the unchanging Knower who watches all of these changes come and go. This Knower is infinite, immortal, and unchanging, the underlying essence of all states of existence, consciousness, and bliss.
- If you notice that your mind has wandered from the repetition of Amaram Hum Madhuram Hum, begin to repeat it once again without thinking that anything wrong has happened.
- Remain sitting and repeating Amaram Hum Madhuram Hum with eyes closed for as long as you feel comfortable.
- When this period of meditation is complete, open your eyes slowly. Be aware that the space which you were perceiving inside and the space which you are now perceiving outside are one and the same.
- If you continue your practice of meditation, your awareness will certainly mature into the Vision of Oneness, the totally free state of consciousness. So meditate for at least ten minutes in the morning and ten minutes in the evening and enjoy the results.

Daily Affirmations

1. **I AM MOTIVATED & ENTHUSIASTIC:**

   I AM Making goals with plans to fulfill them and review them daily.

2. **I AM PROSPEROUS & GIVING:**

   I AM Expecting the best and give without expectation of getting.

3. **I AM COURAGEOUS:**

   I AM Taking risks so that I will grow spiritually.

4. **I AM RESPONSIBLE:**

   I AM Responsible for all I have created in my life, I am not a victim.

5. I AM HEALTHY:

I AM Eating a plant based diet and exercise regularly.

6. I AM GRATEFUL:

I AM grateful for all the blessings in my life and thank God daily for them.

7. I AM FORGIVING:

I AM Seeing all people as innocent children of God in search of love and acceptance.

8. I AM TRUSTING AND TRUSTWORTHY:

9. I AM Understanding that everything that happens in my life is for my best good.

I AM KIND:

I AM Serving.

10. **I AM** LOVING & LOVABLE:

I AM Accepting and empathetic to everyone my life touches.

11. **I AM** JOYFUL:

I AM Following my inner guidance to fulfill my purpose.

12. **I AM** PEACEFUL OF MIND & INTUITIVE:

I AM Praying and meditating every day.

CHAKRAS

Copyright 1995 Susan Boles. Used with permission. All rights reserved. Edited by Dr. Brian Bailey

Chakras and the aura have been studied by Eastern culture (mainly buried in Hinduism) for over 5,000 years. We are more than our physical bodies. We do not end at our skin. Rather our physical body is the densest part of our personal energy. One belief is that our physical body is actually formed around energy spirals called chakras. These energy spirals attract other atoms and coalesce into a solid state through the slowing of their atomic vibration.

The Chinese have mapped the passage of this energy, called Chi, in a system of meridian lines. The human body is criss-crossed with these lines. When 21 meridian lines meet, a major chakra is formed. When 14 meridian lines meet, a minor chakra is formed. Chakras are spinning vortices that enable energy to flow in and out of the physical body.

Each chakra is responsible for the organs near it, and the emotional/spiritual aspects traditionally assigned to it. It is this system that allows us to examine what lessons we need to learn. Illness is a physical manifestation of blocked energy that has its root in our thoughts about ourselves and our world. Illness cannot be "cured" by treating the symptoms as modern western medicine would have us believe. Illness is a compilation of personal beliefs and their related emotions. These beliefs are encoded in the chakras and can cause blockages in the flow of energy. There are different types of blockages but the result is the same. **Beliefs that are causing emotional damage = chakra blocks = illness.**

There is a disturbing current belief that we alone are responsible for our illness or emotional instability. The term responsibility needs to be defined. We are accountable to our bodies for what happens to them; no-one else does as much damage to our bodies as we do. This has its root cause in the scientific community judging our bodies as mere machines, not as the wondrous works of art and soul they are. That is a subject of much greater scope than this discussion will allow.

We often fail to understand the imprint of the generations preceding us. The soul's quest for experience can also be looked at from an archetypal stance. Responsibility is not blame. A lot of newly spiritual people make the mistake of transferring the blame from others to themselves. There is no blame when we are where we are supposed to be in the eyes of our soul. Responsibility means we are the captain of our lives. The soul is the captain. The crew is our bodies, beliefs, our very cells that carry racial/generational memory. The crew has to be trained to go in the same direction so that a certain goal/destination may be reached. Most of us are at cross-purposes with our soul, ignoring those tiny urges and voices until the soul demands you listen. When illness strikes, your soul is trying to teach you something.

Another definition of responsibility is the art of listening to yourself. **Trust your soul and your body.** They alone know what you need—not a book, the newest therapy/therapist, the latest food fad or psychic. All of the former are tools we can use to access our own soul. Responsibility means having power—the power to, not the power over. Allow your soul to have power. It knows how to wield it properly and efficiently without the ego involved.

In the beginning of this allowing the soul power, you may feel a distinct soul/body split. The body is the vehicle for the soul. We need to treat our body as a temple, worshipping it as an integral part of the life experience. To maintain the view that our bodies are machines at the mercy of the mind is very damaging. To dissect the body and treat each part as separate is to believe in the spiritual and emotional life of the body.

Every cell has a memory, otherwise we would be completely renewed each time the cells regenerate. As we come to trust our soul and comply with it's demands, the body becomes more a temple. The outer starts to reflect the inner. Your body reflects what you ingest. True health is the inner light that shines through when you are "conscious." Conscious means spiritually aware, living in the light, aware of responsibility. It is not easy. To be conscious and living the way your soul requires is the highest path here on our planet. Many times when going through a particularly difficult time, I look at the vast majority of humanity who blithely walk through life and wonder "is it all worth it?" Then in a true Celestine Prophecy fashion, a friend tells me a story. "Already having had a traumatic childhood, this monk was horrified to be told by his Master that his life would continue to be difficult. 'Why is God punishing me? I must have done something terrible in a past life to deserve this!' he moaned at the Master. His Master smiled and said, "When a smith puts a rod of steel in the forge, does the steel think it is being punished?" That certainly put my "Why me's" to rest. (For now!)

For every physical disease, there is corresponding emotional unease. Treat the two together to become whole. To heal means to become whole. If your shoulders are sore, what burdens are you carrying that maybe you should release? Taken this simplistically, the symptoms often disappear for a short time. This holds true for many of the physical therapies available. I am a proponent of massage, shiatsu and craniosacral therapy. These therapies are wonderful for the mechanical problems we may have, however, if the problem is rooted in blocked energies caused by outdated beliefs, the relief will be temporary. There is a need to look deeper at the reasons behind the dis-ease. This is the path to understanding and finally putting to rest the reason for the illness. I personally know a woman who reversed ovarian cancer by looking at her beliefs about her body and her life. By connecting with her soul, she reversed the damage. **Never underestimate the power of your soul/body connection.**

Understanding the chakra system allows further scope in understanding what our soul/body is trying to tell us. Every chakra deals with specific parts of our bodies, master glands, as well as emotional specifics. All the chakras are linked to one another through meridian lines. If you are experiencing blockages in one, the surrounding two chakras will also be affected. All chakras are lodged in the spine with front and back aspects except for the root and the crown. The front chakras deal with feelings and the back deal with ego issues. I will list the seven major chakras and their attributes below. The only minor chakras I work with on a regular basis are those in the palms of the hands which connect to the heart, and those behind the knees, which relate to childhood issues.

> *To clarify Susan's chapter I have created a table and drawn a picture, see the end of the chapter, pg. 98-99.*

1. Root Chakra—Color Red—Earth

Located at the base of the spine, this chakra deals with our right to be here. We have the right to food, shelter, love, a clean environment. It is survival. If any of these are not met, we deal with them until they are. Outward manifestations of an upset in this chakra are obesity, sciatica, knee pain, many fears, inability to get and keep a job, inability to form close relationships, money problems. The lesson here is to become grounded in the Earth. Spiritual people become spacey because of concentrating on higher levels of consciousness and forgetting they are human.

Connecting with the Earth like the North American Indians do, will aid here. When meditating, run the energy down instead of up. When walking, feel your feet push into the earth making a solid connection. Wearing red, eating red foods, bathing with a red color lamp and wearing stones like garnet, bloodstone, hematite are helpful.

2. Sexual or Sacral Chakra—Color Orange—Water

Located in the genital area just below the belly button, this chakra deals with our feelings. It is our sexuality and our emotions towards others. We seek pleasure here. From the root chakra, notice others. We reach out to them for information for change and growth. If we learn fear here through inappropriate uses of sex or change, this chakra closes down. Manifestations of upset are sexual addiction or lack of sexual drive, inability to relate to others, emotional neediness or a complete shutdown of emotional response. The water element is beneficial here. Walking near it, swimming, taking baths and showers, just listening to it on tape is good. Wearing orange, eating orange food, using a lamp with a orange color filter, wearing stones such as coral and carnelian are helpful.

3. The Solar Plexus or Will Chakra—Color Yellow—Fire
Located in the stomach, this chakra deals with our views of control, power, our place in the world, government, banking institutions, and our sense of purpose. It is here that we first start to work on our consciousness. **To be conscious is to be in control and know what our purpose is.** We take responsibility for ourselves and change our view from one of victim or blame to one of being co-creator of our lives. If we have been raised with a sense of shame of who we are, the chakra closes down. Outward manifestations of this show up as the need to be in control, excessive anger, an inability to slow down (lack of control), low energy, giving your power to others and addiction to abusive substances. Trouble with the digestive system happens here as this chakra resides over the stomach. Here we feel butterflies when we are nervous. Culturally, this is where we stand.

People are questioning more and more. This is the beginning of our culture moving into the heart vibration. It is called the Fourth Dimension. The heart chakra is the fourth level. Look at the element of fire and allow yourself to be transmuted in the flame. The first three chakras deal with the ego and the element of fire forges our ego to be ready for the enlightenment ahead of us. Wearing yellow, eating yellow food, using a lamp with a yellow filter, and wearing stones such as topaz and amber are helpful.

4. The Heart Chakra—Color Green—Air

Located over the heart, this chakra deals with love and relationship with our world. Here we experience unconditional love for self and others. We learn to balance our male and female sides, our relationships with our mates and our community. We develop compassion (do not read pity here), and self-acceptance. It is here that we see for the first time that we are not alone in the universe. The astral planes make their entrance here. This love is different than in the second. The second is one of finding oneself through merging with another and taking that change into oneself. Here we feel love for all that is. We leave the ego behind and start our learning of things spiritual. We are comfortable with who we are and our place in the world. Now we start to expand into the spiritual realms. We are turning inward to understand ourselves more. This is where our culture is heading. Those of us who are already living in the fourth dimension are seeing that the controls of the third do not work anymore. We are striving to become a global community and work toward the coming of age of our planet. Yet she can't do it unless we do it first for we are her children and she needs us to help her grow.

The element of air shows us how important breathing is. Most of don't know how to breath properly. When we reach this lesson, the desire to heal becomes important. Healing through energy starts here in the heart. There are meridian lines that run from the heart down the backs of the arms and exit through the minor chakra points in the palms of the hands. This heart energy is what heals others. By pooling the energy in our hearts and then pushing it down to the hands, we can affect the energy surrounding a person. As illness is present in the aura before it reaches the physical body, there is a chance of averting the illness. Outward manifestations of blockages in this chakra are inability to love from a non-ego standpoint, codependency, depression, a sense of loneliness and a lack of connection to life. Most of humanity on the planet do not reach this chakra lesson. They are stuck in the third. The Hundredth Monkey Effect[43] is in play however and more and more people are waking up. Wearing green, eating green food, using a lamp with a green filter, and wearing stones such as rose quartz or emerald and malachite are helpful.

5. The Throat Chakra—Color Blue—Ether/Sound

Located at the base of the throat, this chakra deals with communication. It is how we express ourselves, how we communicate with others. Taking this further, we see that creativity resides here. We start to become aware of sound and how it affects us and others. We see how we communicate verbally, how we write. Sound is a purification of our bodies. The Indians tell us that the world was made when God spoke. Sound carries distinct vibrations that can create matter as well as destroy it. When we are "in tune" with a person, it means that we have found a sympathetic vibration; we are on the same wavelength. This is true communication. By listening to beautiful music, we start to unleash more of our soul. By tapping into our creativity in whatever form—playing music, drawing, sculpting, needlework, writing, singing, we start to fine-tune our vibration for the entrance of greater spiritual influence. Many cultures purify themselves before a religious rite by chanting. Develop and chant your own mantras. The opposite of speaking is listening. Develop your listening skills. Outward manifestations of blockages in this chakra

---

[43] Editor's note: The hundredth monkey effect was written about by Ken Keyes in *The Hundredth Monkey,* in it he describes a phenomenon observed by scientists. Observing monkeys a scientist discovered that one monkey learned that washing sweet potatoes made them taste better. This monkey taught its mother and friend until one day 99 monkeys knew to wash their sweet potatoes. The next day when the hundredth monkey learned how to wash its sweet potatoes, an amazing thing happened—the rest of the colony knew how to wash their sweet potatoes too!

Keyes applied this to humankind and explained that when the "millionth" person realizes they can make a difference the whole world will miraculously change.

are the inability to communicate well, lack of creativity, inability to change ways of doing things, sore throats, stiff and sore shoulders, inability to cry or laugh well. Wearing blue, eating fruit, using a lamp with a bright blue filter and wearing stones such as turquoise and blue calcite are helpful. Fill your home with beautiful music and wonderful smells.

6. The Third Eye or Ajna Center Chakra—Color Indigo—Light

Located between the eyes, this chakra deals with the ability to see clearly, the ability to see beyond what our eyes tell us. It is our imagination, our perception of our world, intuition and clairvoyance. Clairvoyance is the ability to see beyond the current reality, to see the aura and the messages it holds for us both about the future and our present. Other spirit is visible. Our memory resides here. It is how we know that a stove is hot. The test here is to go beyond what we normally perceive and stretch our limits further. It is seeing the picture with new eyes. Our memory is very selective. Bad relationships are not all that bad in retrospect, abuse and trauma are often completely blocked from our memories. To look at it may cause shut-downs in other areas of our bodies. We can often predict our own futures by looking at how we are reacting today. If something doesn't change, we will live that future. This is the problem with predicting futures. They are all probable as a conversation with one person can change that future.

Dreams can lead us surely into discovering what our soul requires us to do. Dream books cannot help you. Dreams are very personal and the symbology in them cannot be determined by taking those symbols apart from the dream. Start a dream journal and look for patterns that interweave through your dreams. Using light and color is important in balancing not only this chakra but all the others. Each chakra is given a color and meditating on and running these colors through your body will aid in their balancing. When people are first starting to meditate, the group will be divided into those who visualize and those that sense. Just because you do not "see" objects or colors, yet sense they are there, does not mean that you are doing anything wrong. People who visualize have their roots in Atlantis. People who sense have their roots in Lemuria. I do not visualize but, I can tell you exactly what I sense in terms of objects and colors. It is this ability that allows me to walk into a room and sense others emotions and thoughts. It took a long time to get over that—I was one of the minority who couldn't "see." Outward manifestations of blockages in this chakra are headaches, migraines, inability to correctly interpret what you see, inability to see underneath the visual situation. Wearing indigo, using a lamp with an indigo filter and wearing stones such as lapis, and special quartz crystals for the aid of seeing are helpful. There aren't any foods related to this as it is such a high vibration.

7. The Crown Chakra—Color Violet or White—Thought
Located at the top of the head, this chakra deals with awareness, learning, thought. It is our direct connection to divinity, our higher self, our soul, God/Goddess or all that is. We ask the questions: How we learn? How do we come to get our beliefs? How do we connect to the spiritual world around us? Our beliefs about our world and our place in it emanate from here. The individual chakras then take those beliefs and store them. To transform these limiting beliefs, we need to bring them back up into the crown. From this expanded thought, we can see them for what they are and make the decision to not allow them to affect our lives anymore. The best way to do this is through meditation, and the help of a skilled therapist who will guide you through the situations that birthed those beliefs.

The original belief still resides in us. Our brain is much like a computer in the way it stores memory and the patterns in which we operate. What we are doing in therapy is, in effect, creating another subroutine in the program. When you are faced with a situation that you are trying to change your belief about, you have two ways to approach it—the old routine or the new pathway. It is your choice. One of the best ways to exercise this chakra is to expand our conscious by learning new ways to think, to perceive our universe and to take what is right for us and incorporate it into our daily lives.

Spirituality is very individual and not one path works for all people. Read and experience everything you can and then weed out what does not feel comfortable for you. **Remember that people who try to tell you that their way is the best, are operating from the third level of awareness—control.** We will all get to the point for our soul's maximum learning as long as we don't get in it's way! Outward manifestations of blocked energy in this chakra show as depression, boredom, life is not worth living attitude, inability to learn new things and getting stuck in old programming. People who are excessive about the mind and leaving the body behind become intolerant of others physical problems, their heads are always in the clouds. This viewpoint is in direct contrast with the standard method of enlightenment. The Yogis of before would have us subjugate our bodies to the mind. The lower three chakras were to be brought into strict control and all of the emphasis was put on the upper four. Now we know that we have to live on this planet as humans. We need the first three chakras in healthy order before we can begin to explore the rest of them. Otherwise we will be constantly pulled into the lessons we need to learn. Wearing white or violet, using a lamp with a violet filter and wearing stones such as crystals or amethyst will help. Meditation is of primary importance here.

In conclusion, I hope this sheds some light on the reasons we carry illness and emotions in different parts of our bodies. This is only the tip of the lesson. This life is an illusion, we are not only as we appear. Our task is to grow and develop our souls. The world is the perfect arena for the process. This sounds all so dreadfully serious stop, don't collect $200, go back to Root chakra or continue on to Heyoka—never take yourself or anyone else that seriously!

This chapter is part of a course designed and written by Susan Boles. Susan is a healer and teacher residing in Toronto, Ontario, Canada. If you would like to use this chapter in a publication, please send a letter asking for permission with the name of the publication and description of where it will be distributed. You can contact Susan at:
7 Queensdale Avenue
East York, Ontario
M4J 1Y1
(416) 469-0238

Chakras are strongly related to light and its vibration. The rainbow goes from the lowest vibration of light, red to orange to yellow to green to blue to indigo and finally to violet. Pure white light has all of these. Chakras start at the deepest physical level red and progress to the highest spiritual level of violet.

Three Physical Chakras

1. Root Chakra, red, earth, base of spine, governs the basic physical needs, food, shelter and fight or flight responses.
2. Sacral chakra, orange, water, genital area, governs relationships, sex, pleasure and creativity.
3. Solar plexus, yellow, fire, stomach area, governs sense of purpose and personal power

Four Spiritual Chakras

4. Heart chakra, green, air, heart, governs love, higher self and spiritual connection.
5. Throat chakra, blue, sound, throat, governs expression, communication and judgment.
6. Third eye, indigo, light, between eyes, intuition or spiritual nature.
7. Crown chakra, violet or white, top of head, connection with God.

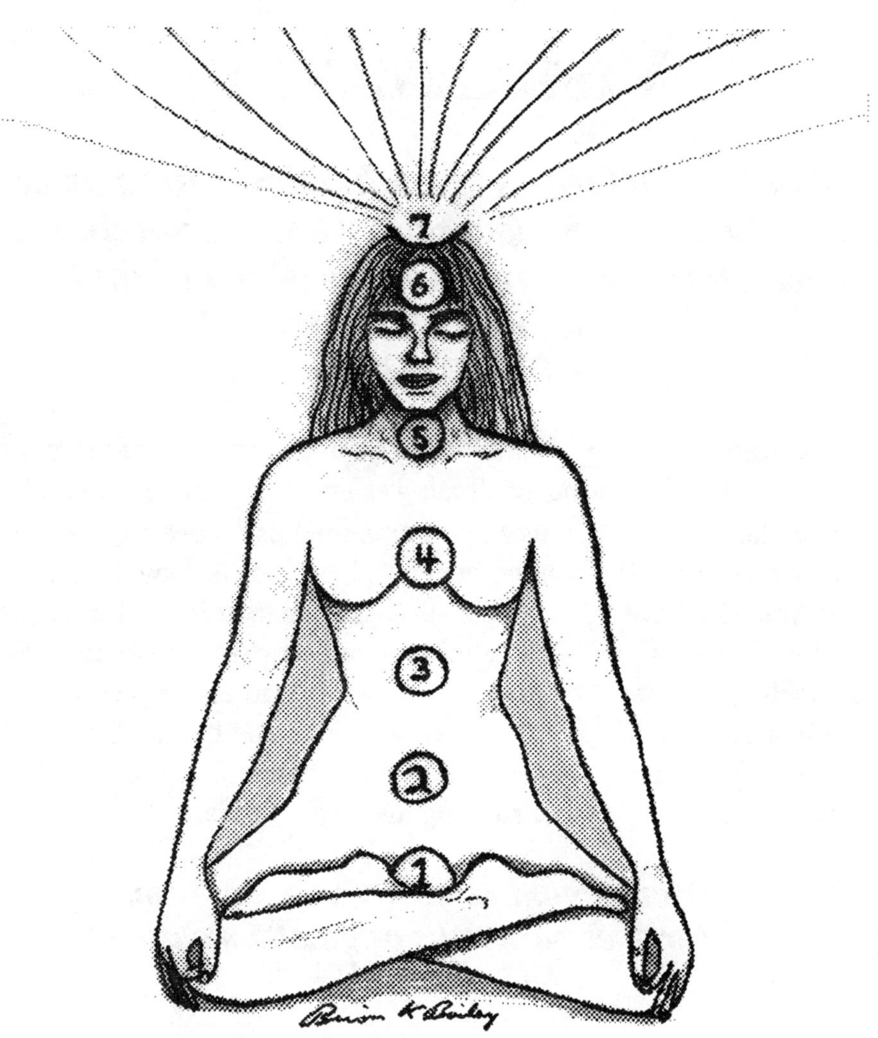

VISUALIZATION

"What lies before us and what lies behind us are small matters compared to what lies within us. And when we bring what is within out into the world, miracles happen."
—Henry David Thoreau

Visualization is a "mind tool" that you can use to "re-program" your mind. It is a kind of "brainwashing." Throughout our lives experiences have taught us and programmed us.[44] Because of these experiences we have formed beliefs. These beliefs may be true or not. We may have false beliefs such as, I cannot do well in school or I can't find a job. This belief is based on past experiences. For example poor performance in school or learned helplessness. I know a 12 year old girl that is very pretty; she thinks she is ugly because of "inner programming." Visualization can erase and re-write these negative tapes running inside our heads.

"Man's mind, stretched to a new idea, never goes back to its original dimension"
—Oliver Wendall Holmes

Visualization creates belief, belief that can alter the circumstances of your life. Visualization means creating pictures in your mind. With visualization, you "speak" directly to your subconscious mind, by-passing the censorship of the left-brain. Your subconscious mind "thinks" in pictures. You can reach the programming levels of your subconscious mind quickly and easily with visualization. Visualization is an idea, a thought form, in picture. By starting with a picture, you take a short-cut directly

---

[44] See chapter Who Am I?

into your right-brain. No words have to be "translated" from left-brain to right-brain language. You deliver a simple, clear, direct message to your subconscious mind.

Real lasting changes in our lives cannot occur until we change our inner person.

Creating visualizations of the things you want to believe is very effective. Your subconscious mind does not rationalize. It takes whatever you give it as "truth." If you consistently picture yourself as having already achieved your goal, your subconscious mind soon believes that it is so. Then, in order to balance your inner and outer reality, your subconscious sets things into motion. The subconscious mind will help create any events or circumstances necessary to produce in the physical realm that which you believe in your mind to be true. Visualization is a bit of mental "trickery." You are, in effect, tricking your subconscious into believing that an event has occurred when it has not. Then your subconscious, seeming to have "fallen behind on the job," gets to work to bring inner and outer reality into alignment. The fact that you only "imagined" the outcome of your goal does not matter. In your right brain (as in space) there is no past, present, or future. Just because you pictured having achieved your goal before you did it, does not matter to your subconscious. If you can make the scene real, you can believe in it. And once you believe in it, it tends to come true.

As within, so without.

We don't have to understand how visualization works, we just have to know that it does work. Numerous studies have been done on visualization, assessing its effect on the performance of athletes, on the ability of students to recall information, and its effect on certain healing processes. From these studies and from the experiences of countless people, we have evidence of the powerful role that visualization can play in our lives. The fact that we don't fully understand it shouldn't stop us from giving it a chance to work for us. We don't fully understand how electricity works, but that does not stop us form turning on the light when we enter a room. So it is with mind tools like affirmations, expectations and visualization. Through experience we can come to predict that they will work for us, even though the universal laws that make their power available to us may not be understood for years to come.

Act as if and fake it till you make it.

The key, then, to using visualization effectively is to make the pictures, the scenes in your mind real. Add all the color, action, energy, and emotion you can muster to the movies in your mind. The more they appear and feel real to you, the more certainly you are creating their (future) reality. In the beginning the movie may be very small, faint and black and white. With your mind you can turn up the sound, size and color each time you play it. The more powerful it is the more effective it will be in changing your life.

> *"We become what we think about all day long."*
> —Ralph Waldo Emerson

Visualization means putting pictures in your mind. For example, try to think of what you had for dinner last night. Think back over the previous evening. What were you doing around dinner time? Who was there with you? Imagine yourself sitting at the dinner table. Look down at your plate. What do you see?

> *"Imagination is more important than knowledge."*
> —Albert Einstein

When you do this, you are visualizing, or creating a picture in your mind. Visualizing helps you remember things. This is because memories are placed into our brains in picture form. But these are not flat, one-dimensional photos—memories are more like moving pictures, complete with all the action, thoughts and feelings that were associated with the original event. By giving your mind a "cue" that hints at the original memory you can bring forth forgotten information. You simply look back over the "movie" in your mind until your see what you need. In a science called neurolinguistic programming, past negative events can be erased by replaying them in your mind and turning down the sound, size, color and emotion. These old movies can even be "taped over" much like a VCR. This technique is used to replace events real or imagined that have created negative thinking or beliefs. Once the old movie is erased, a new positive one can be taped over it. The brain is like a computer disk, if the data is deleted it remains on the disk and can be recovered until it has been written over.

Often, especially in our childhood events may not need to be erased, they may only need editing. Perception of an event eg. a mistake may be perceived as "I am a failure." This perception can be edited to "Wow, that was a powerful lesson!"

Memories are one form of visualization. We all have memories, so we all visualize. But some people visualize better than others. For some people, who are naturally highly visual, creating pictures in their minds comes quite easily. For others, who may be more oriented toward the auditory (hearing) or kinesthetic (feeling) states, visualization takes more practice.

"What we achieve inwardly will change outer reality."
—Otto Rank

Why would anyone want to practice visualization? Because visualization can do much more than bring forth memories. Visualization can be creative, forming original pictures in your mind, pictures that you choose to put there. Earlier I stated that visualization is a bit of "mental trickery." It is this use of visualization that gives you the ability to create your own reality. Remember, inner and outer realities always want to match up. Once an idea is real in your mind (inner reality), it tends to be created in 3-dimensional (outer reality). The trick is to make the thought real in your mind, to truly believe in your creation.

> ***"Change your thoughts and you change your world."***
> —Norman Vincent Peale

This is where visualization can help. "Seeing is believing" for most people. We believe what we see with our own eyes. The same holds true for mental "seeing." Visualizing a scene in your mind tends to make it more real. You come to believe in the reality of the image. At first visualization of a goal may seem forced and unnatural. But repeated visualizations, like repeated affirmations, slowly create the belief that the desired goal is possible, then probable, then finally, a fact. Once a goal has become real in your mind, once you believe it, it starts to become real in your life.

Using affirmations and visualization together is like a "double whammy" for creating belief in your desired goal. One or the other alone will work, but by using the two together, your success will come easier and faster. Visualize your desired goal while you repeat your affirmation for it. Create a scene in your mind where you see yourself already having achieved your goal. See yourself doing what you would be doing, saying what you would be saying, feeling what you would be feeling. By making your visualization vivid, active and exciting you add energy to it.

> ***"As you think so shall ye be"***
> and
> ***"The Kingdom of Heaven is within you."***
> *Jesus*

STEP BY STEP TO BETTER VISUALIZATIONS

Visualization is a process.; it can be made better; it can be honed to perfection. The better you become at visualization, the more creative energy you will have available to create your desired reality.

Start by visualizing in the proper place. Close your eyes and "look" inside your mind. What do you see? Total blackness, of course. Now start to imagine a scene in your mind, perhaps your dinner scene again. Where in your head is this scene taking place?

For many people, visualizations are pictured somewhere in the area of the forehead, often right between the eyebrows. While this is OK, it is more effective to move your mind-movies out away from your head. Picturing your scene between your eyes takes more concentration because your eyes instinctively follow your inward gaze. It is better to move your mind's movie screen out a foot or more from your face, out into space. This allows you to relax more and to have more spontaneous, creative images.

Close your eyes and imagine a movie screen (or if you prefer, a blackboard) a foot or more away from your face and up a couple inches above your eyes. This is where you should make your mental pictures.

First practice making mental pictures with some simple exercises. Imagine (or "draw") on your screen or blackboard a geometric figure, a square, circle or triangle. Keep visualizing this figure over and over for about twenty seconds. Each time your mind wanders, simply bring it back, reproducing the same image over and over. Repeat this exercise with the other two geometric figures.

Then imagine on your mental screen or blackboard a familiar person. You do not need to get details. (Most people don't really see details like hair and eyes on their figures.) In fact, when you "see" an image or visualization, it is in the form of a thought-picture, a sort of mix between an actual image and just the thought of that image. Don't expect pictures like those on television. Trying too hard to get a "good" visualization will hamper your results. Sometimes you "sense" an image more than you actually see it.

Now scan your figure with your mental eye. Note the size, shape and sex of the mental body. Note any feelings or impressions you have about it. Then imagine this body slowly starting to become active, and to move. It might start to walk, jog or play basketball, whatever.

Next, bring another figure into the picture. On your mental screen, see a second figure interacting with the first. Have them talk, shake hands, become animated and argue or laugh together. Practice creating pictures in your mind until you can comfortably imagine and visualize many types of scenes. Creating your own vivid scenes is the key to using visualization. Practice these simple exercises until you become a "natural" at visualization.

VISUALIZING SPECIAL GOALS

While you are making your daily affirmations, you can enhance them with specific visualizations.

Visualizations for Health—Picture yourself on your mental screen, at your healthy best. Imagine yourself strong, vital and healthy as you make your health affirmations.

If there are any areas in your body that need attention, imagine each area specifically, seeing it whole, complete and healed of whatever ailment it once had. Make an affirmation that the ailment is now healed. Imagine a healing light permeating every cell of the affected area. Then, see yourself joyfully experiencing freedom from this ailment. Move the body part freely, breathe deeply, to show that the body part is no longer affected. End the visualization by giving thanks for your perfect health. You can also do these visualizations for others, imaging them on your mental screen.[45]

---

[45] See the chapter: Prayer.

Dr. Bernie Siegel has healed hundreds of patients diagnosed with terminal cancer through visualization. Dr. Siegel spends time with his patients to learn about the type of imagery they use. He has them draw pictures of the disease and how they are going to beat it. He uses these to help the patient use the mind to heal the body. Example: "She saw the tumor as a block of ice, and her therapy and spirituality as warm sunshine entering her body. The tumor essentially melted away." Dr. Siegel has had children use their imaginations to come up with dragons and armies to destroy the disease.

In my own experience, I have seen children destroy a painful wart with imagery. They draw a picture of their foot and the painful wart on the sole of their foot; they put a big red X through the wart and then burn the picture. This treatment works well for children because they "believe." It says in the Bible "Faith can move mountains." Dr. Siegel has documented several cases in which terminal patients were healed simply by faith and belief.[46]

All things existed as thoughts, before their physical reality.

Visualizations for Prosperity—See yourself experiencing your wealth. What kinds of possessions would you have? What would your bank statement look like? Visualize yourself using and enjoying your prosperity. Also, (and this is very important) visualize the good that can come from your increased prosperity.

Perhaps you have plans to help others in some way. Visualize this happening. Any time you use your increased prosperity to help others, you increase your potential for prosperity becoming a permanent part of your life. Your attitude about prosperity and plenty increases your wealth. Think of money as freedom, as a tool to help you do what you do best.

---

[46] See the chapter: Belief: The Power Of Positive Thinking.

You do not have to give away money to use your increased prosperity. If, for instance, your increased wealth allows you to hire help to do jobs that you once had to do, this too, can bring good to others. If you hire a person to clean your house, or someone to mow your lawn. They benefit from income and you have more free time and energy. Now ask yourself, "What will I do with this time and energy?" Will you use it selfishly, thinking only of yourself? Will you use it to serve a higher purpose? or will you use the time to do what you do best to help others?[47]

Perhaps there is a special job or volunteer work that you have been wanting to do, but didn't. Use your prosperity wisely, and more will come to you. Think of your wealth as freedom, security, and added power to help others. When you want to create prosperity, attitude is everything.

Have an attitude of gratitude.

Visualizations for Success—Picture your success in specific, positive images. See yourself performing a service of your choice that others need and appreciate. See yourself being congratulated and praised for your good work. Imagine that you have a never-ending supply of people who value and want your services. See yourself enjoying your work, feeling proud and happy that you can provide this worthwhile service.

If you are not happy with your present job, see yourself working and doing the kinds of things you would really like to be doing. Imagine yourself in the type of environment where you feel the best—at home, at the office, outside, working alone, or working with others. Then give thanks for this new and wonderful job (you do not have to know exactly what this job is—you can leave that up to the universe). See yourself depositing a paycheck into your

---

[47] See the chapter: Finding Your Purpose.

bank account. This check shows the amount of money that you need and desire from your work.

Visualizations for Happiness—Imagine having no wants or needs unfulfilled in your life. Affirm that you already have these things in your life as you visualize them.

See yourself and your loved ones interacting in loving, pleasant ways. Visualize a peaceful scene where your best wishes have come true. Give thanks for the happiness in your life.

There are unlimited ways to visualize. Make your visualizations unique and real according to your own desires. Always remember to visualize the positive outcome of your goal. Visualize the good that will result from having achieved your goal. Visualize yourself being appreciative and thankful. The universe likes to be thanked!

Visualizations for Emotional Healing—Not only can you "program" goals and desires with your visualizations, you can "re-program" old hurts and change old non-productive, limiting attitudes. Using visualization for emotional healing is something that you can do alone if you are committed to looking deeply and openly into your own mind. You can probably successfully use visualization and the other techniques described in this book on your own to help you positively transform your emotional state.

If your scars are buried deeply, or related to a traumatic event, seek professional help in facilitating your personal transformation. If you are too upset to work with a visualization, or get "stuck" and nothing seems to work, you might have gone as far as you can alone. There is nothing wrong with seeking help from qualified professionals for your mental and emotional life. Use your intuition to guide you.

For most people, however, visualization can be a real tool in helping them uncover and re-program their own mental patterns.

The Small Child Visualization—is especially good for re-programming very old beliefs and attitudes. In it you "meet" yourself as a child. You go back to an old feeling or problem and mentally visualize its solution. Even if you don't know the exact problem, by tapping into anxieties, fears or negative feelings, you can get in touch with the mental program associated with them and change them. Go through the visualization several times, each time dealing with a new problem or feeling. A difficult problem may take several repeated visualizations to clear out all the negative energy associated with the original mental program. Follow your intuitive feelings. They will tell you when you have repeated a visualization enough times, or if a sense of peace comes over you during the visualization, or you experience the cessation of a specific anxiety.

> *"Some men see things as they are and say, Why? I dream things that never were, and say, Why not?"*
> —George Bernard Shaw

WHO AM I ?

"Experience is not what happens to a man. It is what a man does with what happens to him."
—Aldous Huxley

The essence of a person is their spirit or soul. This is the real person, not what they seem to be. Before birth we begin receiving input and programming. Programming is the data (experiences) we receive from our **perceptions** of the world. These experiences create memories from which we judge future experiences. Memories create desires which lead us to action.

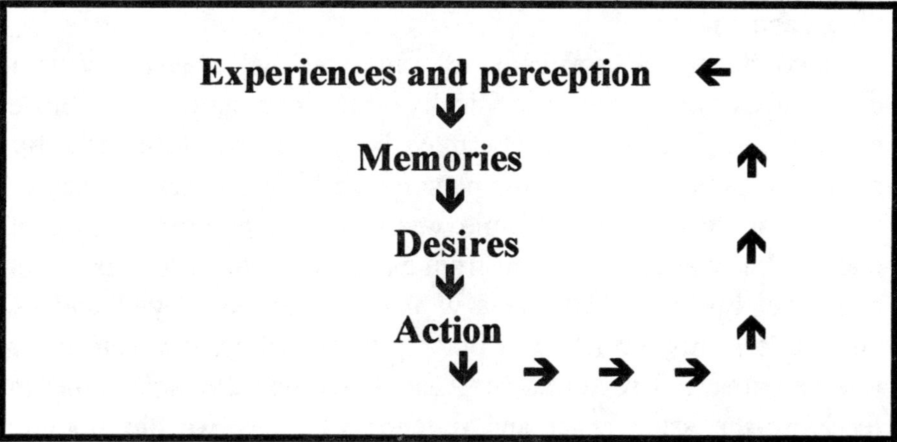

If we only follow our programming, we become victims of our experiences. Some people get stuck in an endless loop of doing the same things over and over again, expecting different results. In a computer this is a freeze, the computer will not respond to input. The computer must be turned off and the program reloaded. If the program won't function with other programs or updates in the system, the program must be updated or rewritten. With humans, we sometimes receive the wrong programming through our experiences or the wrong **perceptions** of these experiences. Most people go through life without ever changing their programming. When they experience freezes such as failed relationships they just start the program over again. People, like computers and jets can crash and burn.

To re-program ourselves, we must access the programmer. The programmer is our center, inner-self or spirit. Our spirit has infinite resources. It has access to the galactic internet or God. Our spirit has no limitations, all possibilities are available. We can change our inner programming through the spirit. Meditate to get in touch with your center. Meditation is similar to quitting all programs temporarily and allowing faulty programs to be repaired, **based on new experiences**. The new experiences that we need are found in books like this, through enlightened counselors and by tapping into the galactic internet.

Once again the software of our soul is created by our experiences or more specifically the perception of those experiences. The same event may be perceived differently by another person or by the same person on a different day because of a different attitude. For example: one of my employees was upset one day because she got a call from a patient's wife who was upset about her husband's bill. This woman proceeded to yell and be very rude to my employee. My employee had her day ruined by this experience. I reviewed the case and called the wife. I began receiving the same anger and rudeness. I knew we did nothing wrong and felt it was blown out of proportion. I asked her what was **really** wrong. At that point she began to cry and tell me how her mother was dying and she was having financial problems. I listened to her for quite some time. She softened and we worked out the problem, and I kept a patient and made a friend. The point here is the perception of the event. My employee felt shame and inadequacy as the result of the wife's anger and rudeness. These feelings were based on her past experiences as a child. When she was a child her parents and some of her teachers would yell at her if she did something wrong. She learned that she was flawed, not good enough. The feeling of toxic shame[48] prevented her from successfully dealing with this problem. The lesson from this example is that our programming can often be a roadblock to our happiness.

How does this all work? Perception of an experience becomes a memory. Memories create desires and desires are the driving force of our actions and thus experiences.

How do we change our programming? We can change our perceptions by thinking from a higher level, a more intuitive level. We can meditate and get in touch with our memories and desires. Our programming is in the subconscious, thus we, are largely, unaware of most memories and desires. To change them we must know them or we will go through life saying, "Now why did I do that?" The worst case scenario of bad programming is called **denial**. Denial is not knowing or realizing what we are doing. The classic example is the alcoholic that beats his wife and children. This man doesn't understand or want to do what he does. He denies it or finds reasons for doing it. The victims are usually in denial too. They make excuses and cover up for him. The wife may have been programmed by her parents to chose that type of mate. If she leaves him and doesn't change her programming she will most likely do it again.

Can we change memories from the past? No, but we can change our perception of what happened. If we look at an adverse event from the past we can look through our more intuitive and empathetic eyes and re-perceive the event. We can forgive, accept and take responsibility for whatever we were responsible for.

Memories and desires create thoughts. We may not be able to prevent negative thoughts, we can cancel them and replace them with positive affirmations. For example, "This kid is driving me crazy!" To, "This child is a real challenge, she will teach me patience and we will grow together."

---

[48] Toxic shame is feeling that I am bad instead of I made a mistake.

Desire is the progenitor to action. If we understand our desires we can control them instead of them controlling us. We can make choices based on **all** our desires and not leap into action based on every little whim and desire.

BEFORE BIRTH/AFTER DEATH?

I have studied many world religions. I have found many similarities. Today, science has unveiled many great spiritual truths—such as the power of the mind to heal the body with prayer, meditation and visualization. Science has opened another realm, life after death. Numerous books have been written about after death experiences. Some scientists have tried to explain it away, saying after life experiences are just the result of brain programming to lessen the impact of death. The evidence is overwhelming, our spiritual life continues after death.

Birth—Our souls are immortal; they are pure energy, similar to light energy. We are all pieces of the divine. Before we are physically born, the soul leaves its home, soulmates and fellow spirits to enter the developing baby's body. Soon the lessons will begin. We chose our life situation with divine guidance to expand our spirituality. No soul can ever learn all it needs to know from one life. We return again and again to this challenging school called Earth life. Unlike the spirit world, we feel alone—we are not alone. We all have one or two guardian angels to watch over us, from now on I will call them guides. Our guides will help to keep us on the learning path we have chosen. Some may not listen to their guides and waste a life experience thus delaying spiritual progression. As I have said so many times before, our guidance comes from deep within ourselves. Our soul knows our mission, our purpose in life, it also knows the subtle clues and hints that are given to us by our guides. We may also receive impressions from those in our soul groups.

Each soul belongs to a special group of souls, a learning group. Every group is at a different spiritual level and has different spiritual needs. The average size of these primary groups are 15 souls. Souls may interact with other groups but they mainly interact with their primary group. The primary group of souls interact frequently on Earth as brother, sister, spouse, close friends and less often as parents or children.

Between Earth lives intense study is done of the former life. What were the choices and possibilities? What lessons did they learn and how might they do things differently in the next life. These experiences are shared with their group. Communication is telepathic so nothing is hidden. Souls are not judgmental or negatively critical, they always have the best interest of each other in mind. Groups have teachers who are at higher levels and are still progressing themselves. Souls use Earth memories to relate with their environment. Their learning area may be seen by one spirit as a modern class room and by another as an open aired Greek temple. Souls will also project images of themselves similar to bodies they have had on Earth.

Soon after the last life was reviewed, a soul may choose to experience another life. The group, teachers and guides help the student/soul to choose the next situation. There are other learning areas for souls in the spirit world, for more information on these read *Journey of Souls (Case Studies of Lives Between Lives)* by Dr. Michael Newton. Dr. Newton has used hypnosis to regress hundreds of people into past lives and more importantly to lives between lives.

An important lesson I have learned is that young spirits are more susceptible to the passions and desires of the human brain and body. They are more self-centered, more violent and generally more spiritually immature. In the past, when counseling patients, at times I couldn't understand why they didn't seem to be able to grasp spiritual concepts. Even though a young spirit is highly intelligent, they have little curiosity about things beyond the physical and concrete (first chakra level). I now can understand, it is because of the lack of experience of these young spirits.

Unfortunately, it is quite unlikely that a young spirit would ever read this book. If you are reading this and learning you are most likely a more advanced spirit. Advanced spirits are more likely to seek out spiritual truths. Advanced spirits are less controlled by passions, emotions and physical desires of the human body. This is not to say these passions, emotions and desires are not present, they are, advanced souls experience them, but are not controlled by them. They have developed their higher chakras. Advanced spirits are more interested in seeking personal truths and assisting in the advancement of the human race either with individuals or on a larger scale. The purpose of this book is to help all souls to learn these vital lessons and help us to make the most of this life. So, what about death?

Death—when we die our spirit separates from our body. It is a tough transition. We are pulled out of our bodies by a force that feels like a magnetic force. We generally float out of our body and observe what is happening. It is difficult for many of us to leave our family and friends behind. We feel the force pulling us up and away. Many spirits resist returning to the spirit world until after the funeral. We then are pulled through what seems to be a long tunnel toward a light. Our guide and often deceased family members or close friends will be waiting to assist in the transition. Traumatic life experiences may necessitate a debriefing before we return to our groups.

Once we are ready, we are eager to return to our groups. We are coming home to those who know us so well and love us unconditionally. We may not be proud of our last life performance because we are our own worst critics. Our group helps us to see unwise choices and learn the lessons that were intended in the lives we have led. We also benefit by the sharing of other's life experiences.

Choosing the next life experience—at this point in our journey there are lessons to be learned, karmic events to be played out and assisting other souls with their learning. When all is balanced, our teachers and higher coordinators give us the choices of new life possibilities. We can see the potentials of these lives and possible futures.[49]

Once our choice is made and we enter a human body we have a destiny, a path to follow. Sometimes traumatic emotional events or bad childhood experiences can prevent us from living our potential if we let it. We may need a good counselor to help us repair the damage to our subconscious mind. Our soul is limited by the human brain. Only partial expression of the soul is possible in humans. A defective brain or damaged subconscious mind will limit our soul's ability to learn. **This may be the plan.** If not, the person will be guided to those who can help.

The purposes of life— are to learn to love, understand and accept all people; to connect with the oneness of all people, places and things. These are very high level goals that are predicated on the learning of the primary lessons. I have tried to include as many of those primary lessons as I could. In the sequel to this book there will be more lessons as well as repeats taken from a different angle or expanded. If you can think of anything that can be added feel free to contact me.[50]

---

[49] The future can only be seen to a limited extent because the future is fluid possibilities are innumerable.
[50] See the end of the book for contact information.

RELIGION

*"the fruit of the spirit"—love, joy peace,
patience, kindness, generosity, faithfulness,
gentleness and self-control.*
—From Galatians 5:22-23

Religion can have either positive or negative effects on a person's life. The true test of whether a religion is good for you or not can be discovered by answering the following questions:

1. Does it teach the fruit of the spirit **or** does it focus on "sin."
2. Does it increase your self esteem **or** do you feel you can never measure up to the "standard"?
3. Are you becoming more loving, accepting and tolerant of people who believe differently than you **or** do you feel that your belief is the only correct path?
4. Are you open to all possibilities **or** is your mind closed to new ideas?
5. Are you increasing your sense of connection with all living beings and Mother Earth?
6. Are you realizing that all negative energy sent out to people places or things actually harms you, while positive energy heals you?
7. Are you following the teachings of men when your spirit whispers no?
8. Do you fear death and judgment or do you believe in a supreme power that wants the best for you?
9. Do you understand that earth life is only a classroom? If we fail, we will not be cast into hell or somewhere else. We may fail over and over, the important thing is that we learn and progress. All we need to do is pay attention and keep on trying.

There are and will be many more great teachers from all over the world and from many different religious backgrounds. The greatest influence in my life is a Teacher who walked the Earth almost 2,000 years ago. He was, in my humble opinion the greatest teacher of all time. His lessons were simple. He taught unconditional love and acceptance of all people. He taught about mistakes, forgiveness, prayer and a lot more.

Despite His message of love and peace His teachings infuriated the religious leaders of His time. These pillars of the community caused Him to be rejected by his own people and put to a horrible death by the government leaders.

If your religion is one that would promote negative thinking by condemning other people, religions or yourself then let it go.

Note: I believe this country is experiencing a spiritual awakening. Angelic encounters continue to grow in number. Eileen Elias Freeman, the author of *Angelic Healing* (Warner Books), collects about a dozen angel stories a week by mail (you can write to her at P.O. Box 1397, Mountainside, NJ 07092) and e-mail, where her address is 70334,300@CompuServe. Joan Wester Anderson, author of *An Angel to Watch Over Me* (Ballantine), which relates "true stories of children's encounters with angels," says she's been getting about 25 letters a week from children alone (Box 1694, Arlington Heights, IL 60006; she can't guarantee a response to every letter).

ANGELS, GUIDES AND GUIDANCE

We have all heard that small still voice within, throughout our lives guiding us. We have all, at times chosen to not listen. The habit of indifference to this inner voice of guidance can become so ingrained, we no longer hear it. Instead, we are satisfied to listen to our conscience, those rules of "civilized" behavior—the litanies of rights and wrongs—by which we self-judge and are judged in a "normal" society.

Conscience is a learned response. It is an evolved capacity of the subconscious mind that holds us back from expressing the spectrum of deepest darkest, negative behaviors. Conscience results from the rule of law.

The capacity for conscience began over 5000 years ago. It is part of the contract of survival for higher levels of civilization, higher populations living together in smaller environments— communities—within the context of a specific belief or religious system. The rule of conscience rather than consciousness in itself sets the stage for dichotomous inner conflicts. It comes out of an authoritarian concept of forced self-control. It breeds cold, logical rule followers, that have no mind of their own.

Acceptable behavior differs from group to group. In power struggles, leadership finds it easy to manipulate the belief systems based on conscience. In our present society, in the struggle for space and for self-identity, this ideal of conscience applied to relationships intimate, familial and regional is no longer valid. Where individual worth is negated, no life is sacred.

The new learning must be in self-love, self-awareness, self-responsibility—consciousness. Only spiritual growth can bring this evolutionary change, for these are qualities of higher states of mind, higher states of being. We are beginning to walk a completely new path of possibility.

The energy of the Awakening is moving into all levels of our beings. The ground rules are shifting, and we are all seeking some kind of leadership in this time of change. The new teachers in higher consciousness rarely come from incarnated[51] humanity, but from beings in the spirit world—our own higher selves and our spirit guides.

Some individuals have long relationships with angels and guides. Others remember a time in childhood when a radiant being was a friend. Others tell stories of angels and visitations by higher beings in moments of duress, stress or trauma. Many individuals are now speaking out about their experiences with these "other-worldly" beings.

Guidance by our higher selves and angelic beings has always been available to us. We have all been persuaded to some extent to the non-existence of the inner voice or the outer voices of guidance. For some of us, to have conversations with these guides is akin to severe mental distress. Many churches teach that contact with God must be though a mediator such as a priest. Religion teaches a separation, an impossibility of knowing or becoming our higher selves in this lifetime. The majority simply disallow these realities entirely.

The spiritual journey is helped by higher beings, spiritual teachers to teach us the ways of unconditional love. We benefit from communication, sources of encouragement, explanation and discernment. Our higher selves and our guides provide all of these and surround us with their unconditional love. They represent the new possibility of who we are to become.

---

[51] Incarnate means to become flesh, it happens when the spirit enters the body.

Spiritual Guidance

We were all sent to Earth with the ability to call home when we need help. This ability lies within our spirit, our very center. To some, it is praying and receiving answers. Perhaps a more precise term is channeling. We are all connected by threads or channels to the spirit world where a piece of our spirit remains. Our connection with home (the spirit world) is through the spirit and then through this channel. Much like a TV channel our spirits have a frequency, a vibration—it is this vibration we must get in tune with to tap into the spiritual realm.

Channeling is born of meditation. Meditation is born of quieting the mind. In training myself and others to communicate directly with the spirit, I have noticed that beginners have more difficulty with emotional and mental stillness than with any other phase of channeling. Why is that so? Some of us have emotional scars and unhealed wounds from childhood and other past experiences. These need to be healed before we can completely connect with the spirit.[52] To begin this healing, find a counselor that understands emotional and spiritual healing. Two tools that can be used for this type of healing are journaling and healing touch.[53]

Once we are in the habit of getting in tune with our spirit then we will be able to communicate with our guides.

Perhaps you have known of a religious community unsettled by reports that channeling is evil. Channeling (communicating directly with God's messengers) is a mystical component in biblical heritage. All religions have a mystical origin. A prophet or shaman experiences direct revelations from spiritual realms. Followers crystallize their revelations into rituals, doctrines, and other disciplines for the masses. Institutional religion flourishes. Divine revelation to individuals seems to vanish. The term "religion" (from the Latin "religare") originally meant "to re-connect or link back."

---

[52] See the chapter Chakras.
[53] See the chapters: Journaling and Healing Touch.

Re-connecting with our spiritual home? Could that include a live, in-the-moment, direct, conscious connection?

The Bible is replete with accounts of direct spiritual communication. It appears that Paul believed direct revelation from "prophetic spirits" was available to many in his flock. He said, "For you can all prophesy in turn." (I Corinthians 14:31) Paul encouraged people at religious meetings to prophesy "so that everybody will learn something and everybody will be encouraged." He said, "Let two or three (prophets) speak. If one of the listeners receives a revelation, then the man who is already speaking should stop ... Prophets can always control their prophetic spirits ..." (I Corinthians 14:30-34) Prophecy was considered a gift of the Spirit. (I Corinthians 12:10-11) Prophesying was also a service: "who prophesies does so for the benefit of the community." (I Corinthians 14:4) These passages reveal the remarkable resemblance between prophesying and spiritually-based channeling.

"The Kingdom of God is within you." (Luke 17:21)

It makes sense that our loving God created us with a built-in way to call Home Base. Consider direct spiritual communication as an innate human capacity to be cultivated with loving intentions, spiritual integrity, and diligence.

Angels/Guides

Much has been written about these ethereal beings. Some call them angels, guardian angels, spirit guides or spirit people. Regardless of the name, these beings are available to us to guide us on our path of life.

A word of caution: many individuals do not realize there are voices that can speak to us from our subconscious mind, these voices are those of past experiences not demons or devils. Voices of parents, teachers or our own internal critics may speak to us.

These voices may be critical, negative and may not have our best interests at heart. Angels, guides and our own spirit speak with unconditional love and acceptance.

In spiritual guidance, each being in incarnation has many guides and teachers, some who have been with us from the first moment we decided to incarnate. We are not strangers to each other. Prior to incarnation in any lifetime, we sit with our guides and decide what our lessons will be, through whom we will learn the lessons, and how we will learn them. If, in any lifetime, we have need of these higher beings, they are there to assist, with empathy and love.

The master teachers in the spirit world come into our minds when we are learning new work or experimenting with new learning. They assist as mentors. When they are no longer needed, they move on and new teachers appear for the newer or higher work or learning. Guides and teachers are also beings on a journey of spiritual growth. They are on a higher level of spiritual growth and are still learning through guiding us. As we advance on our paths, so do they.

Most people believe their angels and guides are invisible. However, there is a great deal in literature on the subject of visibility that shows some individuals are more sensitive to higher vibration than others. Regardless of being able to see them or not, having and knowing of their presence is enough. To be able to converse and debate with them is far more important. The teachings come through one or two-way communication.

As we consciously begin our spiritual journeys, we become aware of these beings. Sometimes they come unbidden into our consciousness. Some of us have been frightened or put off by these ethereal presences. Some people have been carefully programmed by their religion to believe this is part of the "occult" or the forbidden things which we must never acknowledge or allow into our lives. As a result, many of us need to be taught how to open to, connect and communicate with these beings.

When the student is ready, the teacher appears.

It is important to remember that angels/guides will appear to us as beings we can understand and relate to. For one person, a guide will appear as the classic angel with wings and flowing white robes, to another, a guide might appear as an ancient wiseman. For most people, there is only the small, still voice.

Our guides and teachers are there to give us the help we need. They are there to answer any and all questions we have. Their answers come from a perspective that is so much higher than our own. They pull us along into higher knowledge and higher understanding just by the nature of their beings. They show us the paths we are on from past through present and speak to us about the changes we must make to continue on a more peaceful, self-loving spiritual journey.

Many times, what we are being told is not understood in our current state of consciousness. Nevertheless, there are some deep inner changes that take place each time we listen. What they tell us will change us profoundly when we ponder each thought.

Guides exist at higher levels of vibration. They have form, but it is of a more radiant nature. Higher guides have already completed the work of clearing lower issues and are no longer focused on fear. Some of them are still incarnating, while others have finished that phase of learning. They are free from the fear and separation that hold us in physical manifestation. They are with us to teach, and through teaching to learn higher lessons themselves and continue to even higher possibilities.

These beings are here to help us maximize the experiences in this life, use them as much as possible.

One person's description of help from guides

"When I am angry, depressed, unsure, or feel incapable of a forward step, my guides are always there in unconditional love. They show me where my thinking is in error, speak of higher ways of thinking about handling the same situation, help me to have patience with the process of creation, lead me to do what is for my highest good, and help me clear those issues or memories or emotions that bind me to the old ways of thinking and doing.

I have come to trust this higher awareness that is always available to me. These beautiful beings provide solace, come forward to be with me in all times of highest joy and lowest depression. They lead me to those who can most help me and advise against relationships that would distress or deplete me. They bring into my life those who need my help and who form a healing circle of giving and receiving so that I can grow and learn as well from each encounter."

Besides guidance, there are a many things we can do for ourselves to move into higher awareness: read books, listen to tapes that open us to higher truths, develop relationships with individuals already on their higher paths, join groups exploring higher possibilities and learn to meditate, to go inward into a quiet, peaceful state.

Identifying Your Personal Guides

There is no mystery to accepting guidance into our lives. We merely need to allow it. Our higher selves and guides are happy to speak to and work with us. First, we must ask. Then we receive. Don't forget to say thank you.

Many of us come to this time of opening up to guidance with reluctance, doubt and disbelief as to its efficacy and truth. We continue to hear indoctrinated biases and feel an ambiguity or indifference. Our belief systems are shocked to hear realities so extraordinarily different. We are suddenly asked to accept, on faith and with love, the unknown and unseeable.

When we desire spiritual healing, growth and change more than we have ever desired anything else, we are open to receive spiritual guidance from our higher power and our higher selves.

As we put aside our learned biases and willingly open our hearts, we allow a connection to our spiritual guides. Because they are in higher vibration, they need to create pathways, energetic passages, from their level of vibration down to our denser levels.

The lowest or most dense level of vibration they can attain is at the level of the heart[54]...the gateway to the astral planes, the spirit world. We know the connection to higher guidance by the warmth and vibrations we feel in our hearts. We must also know that we are not receiving higher guidance if we do not feel this heart connection.

The first mental contact with guides may feel strange. In the spirit world, all communication proceeds out of thought. All communication is instantaneous and unblocked by negativity. This communication is in the form of symbols, ideograms and images. While our guides are ever listening to our verbalizations, they generally need to shift their communication skills to match ours. With a bit of patience, this readjustment to our level of consciousness is completed. The first communications may be garbled and unclear, coming in at a rate that we cannot handle, much like a computer modem faster than our own. We must tell our guides when we do not or cannot grasp what they are saying so they can continue to adjust to us.

At first, when we recognize the presence of an awareness other than ourselves within our minds. This may feel uncomfortable, an intrusion into our inner beings. The more we have been victimized in our lives, the stronger our control issues, the higher the level of distrust and discomfort in this union of energies. When we trust and have faith this is a being of unconditional love we will be lead us to our highest good, we will feel safe to have this presence join with us.

---

[54] See the chapter: Chakras.

If we ask, guides are usually happy to tell us their personal histories and to give us their names. Guides recently incarnated usually use their previous name. Other guides simply find a name acceptable to our level of consciousness. Other guides never identify themselves by a name, and do not wish to have a humanized identity.

Whether we acknowledge our clairvoyance or not, we all have the ability to receive images and a knowing from outside ourselves. It is the very nature of sensual perception. In our current belief system, we believe we are reacting to and perceiving sensual input from outside of ourselves. In fact, we are the creators of all that unfolds before us. What we perceive with the senses, we have created in our thoughts and are then experiencing in form.

Everything is merely a thought. We are in a constant state of sending out or receiving thought. In a state of unconsciousness, we do not possess this awareness of ourselves. In higher states of awareness, we know the truth of this.

In all communication and interaction, we are processing incoming energy and reacting to it according to our level of awareness. Seeing is merely the outcome of reacting to a burst of light vibration we interpret according to our beliefs about that energy. We receive this energetic input and process it deeply within ourselves on the TV screen of the mind. Likewise, the images remembered from our dreams—our travels in the astral planes and beyond—are not sight or eye images, but images, symbols and visualizations perceived within our inner knowing.

Moving into higher vibration, higher consciousness opens this awareness of the process of thought and visualization. Seeing our guides with our eyes is not necessary for communication. When we are ready to accept higher energy as a reality in our lives, we will move into a knowing the energetic forms of these beings as they exist in higher vibration.

Their importance to us is not in being seen, but as bringers of higher knowledge and wisdom. They can see our totality, are conversant with our own spiritual selves and act as go-betweens for that highest vibrational awareness and our current state of dense vibration.

They see our entire path of light and know the lessons we are learning. Their desire is to move us out of the suffering and into love and joy quickly and easily. Connection to their higher vibrations makes this transition transpire more readily.

As we stretch our perceptions into higher vibrations, we simultaneously open ourselves to more universal energy and to even higher awareness. We are stretching our energy of individual awareness out and connecting with our higher selves, with each other at higher levels.

Forming Relationships With Our Guides

Forming a friendship with our guides is akin to forming any other relationship. We will put them through a time of testing to see if they will really always be there for us. We will question everything they tell us.

While we are still untrusting, we might ignore the advice and teachings and continue to create events and relationships in our lives which cause us pain. When we finally conclude we need to seek help to go higher and become clearer in our lives, we arrive at acceptance and trust for these higher beings and their teachings.

When we remember that our spirit knows the truth of all things we will not be misled. To regularly reconnect to your spirit, make it a habit to meditate at the start of your day and at the end to review your day.

The warmth and love of friendship grows with time and experience. When we feel these beings with us, holding us lovingly in our weak and pained moments, when their advice takes us out of harms way, and when we feel ourselves expanding and changing, we allow ourselves to open to them fully. Their unconditionality brings a new concept into friendship and relationships. Our expectations and perceptions of friendship shift into this new reality.

To know, without doubt, we are surrounded by love is to move into a new level of existence we never dreamed possible. We find we are loved for who we were, who we are, who we will be, our paths, our thoughts, our emotions and our beliefs. Every consciousness shift, every lesson learned is applauded. We are supported through all our hard times. Through their unconditional love we can better learn self love.

They ask nothing from us, but offer us everything they are and know. Through them, we learn an *attitude of gratitude*, a gratefulness for connection with spirit. We also learn gentleness, kindness, caring, sharing openly and fully.

As they bless us, we learn to bless ourselves and others. Through their eyes we begin to see and accept our uniqueness and potential. By accepting these qualities in ourselves we learn to accept and respect the uniqueness and potential of others. Our love and joy is theirs and theirs becomes ours. Our spiritual growth contributes to their happiness and their fulfillment.

A Spiritual Revolution

This world is beginning a spiritual revolution, people are waking up. We have a collective responsibility to help those around us to wake up and live their lives to the fullest.

The Awakening, the Age of Aquarius, began back in the 40's and 50's as people became aware that the old ways were not uplifting. Some of you may remember the consciousness-raising movements of the 50's and 60's, the women's movement, the black movement, the gay rights movement, the whole earth movement, the anti-war movement and the human rights movement.

All of these were designed to lift the human mind out of the deep sleep of the past and to invigorate new possibilities. The 70's and 80's are called a flat time because people began focusing on their own lives. They were moving into awareness of their needs and desires for change out of "old world" beliefs.

Since the later 80's there has been a spiritual awakening. Many of us who are spiritual seekers have been labeled as liberals, New Agers or worse, cult members.

Much of humanity lives desperate lives, caught in an economic and social backlash. The Awakening brings an inrush of energies that stirs the pot of change. We are in a time of emotional desperation for many who will not accept change, but hold to the old authoritarian beliefs.

Fear is everywhere. It is being manipulated masterfully. Chaos, confusion and destructiveness can increase. Fundamentalists are heralding the coming of the End Time, the return or coming of the "True Messiah." We are all exposed to this growing paranoia.

There are many prophecies about the "end time": the Hopi speak of moving to the Fifth World; the Book of Revelations speaks of the apocalypse and the 1,000 years of peace and love to follow; the American Indian traditions predict this time of destruction, depletion and chaos followed by a return to living with the earth; Judaism speaks of a time when the lion will lie down with the lamb; Hinduism points to this as the era of Kali, the goddess of destruction by fire and rebirth into the light.

We who are moving through spiritual self-transformation, and especially healers, are asked to be on the vanguard of this evolutionary step for humankind.

Alternative healing and self-transformation are becoming more "fashionable." However, beware of the charlatans that are "selling" quick-fix approaches as a substitute for the longer process of true self-transformation.

KINDNESS/SERVICE

Commit random kindness,
senseless acts of beauty
—bumpersticker

"If each of you reading this practiced just one
random act of kindness a day, starting tomorrow,
our world would be transformed."
—Barbara DeAngelis, Ph.D.

Kindness, like violence can build on itself, the choice is ours. Do we want to cultivate the seven deadly sins[55] and have them erupt into a mushroom cloud—or do we want to begin a chain reaction with each act of random kindness that blossoms into world peace and love.

Dr. Viktor Frankl a survivor of the Nazi death camps and author of *Man's Search For Meaning.* said, **"Ask not what you can expect of life; ask what life expects of you."** Dr. Frankl discovered that the survivors had a purpose, a meaning for living that was beyond themselves. Two decades later President John F. Kennedy gave this advice in his inaugural address, "My fellow Americans, **ask not what your country can do for you, ask what you can do for your country."** This law of giving and receiving is universal, it is also known as the law of karma; what goes around comes around. Whatever we put into the world comes back to us, particularly when it involves people. If you want to be happy, serve someone to create happiness in their lives. If you want a friend, be a friend. If you want love, give love. If you desire success, then help someone else become successful. The hardest

---

[55] According to St. Gregory "The seven deadly sins are: pride, lust, sloth, envy, anger, covetousness and gluttony."

one to understand is: if you want more money, give more money. This is **the law of tithing**. In Malachi 3:10, God promises the Israelites that if they give their tithes he will open the heavens and pour them "out a blessing, that there shall not be room enough to receive it." A tithe has traditionally meant a tenth of your increase (gross income). A tithe should not be money alone, to get karmic benefits, a tithe should be of your time, talents and resources. Churches often require their members to donate to the church. The church then decides how the money will be spent. I believe it is better for the individual to find a good cause and donate. Giving clothes and food to the poor or helping some poor struggling family. If you are short of money or not, give time. Search your talents and discover how you can best serve your community then do it. The writers of *Chicken Soup for the Soul* accept donations of the price of one book to donate 2 books to prisons, shelters and other needy institutions, I make the same offer with this book.[56]

I don't believe in welfare to the extent that it enables people to be dependent on the government. Wouldn't it be better to give them the training they need to find jobs or even provide community service jobs? Instead of food stamps to buy junk food, wouldn't it be better to give healthy food. Whole grains, beans, vegetables, fruit and surplus foods? The same applies to our children, don't give them everything they want, help them to help themselves or they will remain dependent on you or expect the world to take care of them. As you venture forth to serve, do it well, think what is best, what would you want done for you in the same situation—keep the future in mind.

The Golden Rule:
Do for others what you would have them do for you.

---

[56] Please send names of worthy organizations you may know of. The address for this and donations is in the resource directory.

*Before you criticize and choose, walk a
mile in my shoes.*

> Lord, I am an instrument of thy peace.
> Where there is hatred, I sow love. Where
> there is injury, pardon. Where there is
> darkness, light and where there is sadness
> joy.
> O, divine master, I am thankful that I
> may not so much seek to be consoled, as to
> console; to be understood, as to
> understand; to be loved, as to love; for it is
> in giving that we receive, it is in
> pardoning that we are pardoned, and it is
> in dying that we are born to eternal life.
> —ST. FRANCIS OF ASSISI[57]

**When ye are in the service
of your fellow beings ye are only
in the service of your God.**
—Book of Mormon, Mosiah 2:17

**ONE OF THE BEST CURES FOR DEPRESSION IS
TO HELP SOMEONE, SERVE THEM.**

---

[57] I modified this slightly, I replaced make me an instrument with I am an
instrument and I replaced O, divine master, grant that I with O divine master, I
am thankful that I.

"It's the action, not the fruit of the action that's important. You have to do the right thing. It may not be in your power, may not be in your time, that there'll be any fruit. But that doesn't mean you stop doing the right thing. You may never know what results come from your action. But if you do nothing, there will be no result."

—Gandi

"It is one of the most beautiful compensations of this life that no man can sincerely try to help another without helping himself"
—Ralph Waldo Emerson

Seek to serve others rather than to be served by them. However, don't be so proud that you refuse to accept or ask for help when you need it—you will be denying someone else the opportunity to serve.

TRANQUILLITY—PEACE OF MIND[58]

What is a greater accomplishment in life than serenity and peace of mind? What asset could be of more value to us than unshakable calmness and tranquillity? What better evidence of spiritual strength could we have than a peaceful mind and heart?

Peace of mind comes from accepting what we cannot control and taking responsibility for what we can. It grows out of faith and trust in our Higher Power and our spiritual natures. It comes to us when we let go of our guilt, fear and doubt.

IT IS THE RESULT OF FORGIVING OURSELVES AND OTHERS FOR ALL HUMAN IMPERFECTIONS.

We can learn independence from turbulent emotions and negative thoughts. We can discover that happiness originates inside, not outside, of us. When we let go of our delusion that something or someone will someday make us happy, we can focus on our spiritual center and the joy we have within.

INNER PEACE IS ALWAYS FOUND IN THE HERE AND NOW. IT WAITS QUIETLY FOR US TO DISCOVER IT.

We can turn our conscious minds away from worries, fears, regrets, expectations, and the haste of our daily lives. Then all the love, beauty, joy, and peacefulness of our deep spiritual selves can come through.

Without peace of mind, no amount of wealth or good fortune can ever make us truly happy. With true peace of mind, no adversity or lack can ever disturb our calm soul.

If I had but one wish for everyone, guaranteed to come true, it would be this: That there would be peace and love among all

---

[58] Based on Peace by my old friend Susan Smith Jones.

people, beginning with peace inside each person. There is nothing in the world more valuable than peace and unconditional love. It is within each of us to choose love and peace as a conscious goal.

WHEN WE ARE AT PEACE, WE CREATE AND EXPERIENCE HEAVEN ON EARTH.

Serenity and peace is within you, sit, be still and tune in to the small, still voice within.

DESIDERATA

Go placidly amid the noise and haste, and remember what peace there may be in silence.

As far as possible without surrender be on good terms with all persons.

Speak your truth quietly and clearly; and listen to others even the dull and ignorant; they too have their story.

Avoid loud and aggressive persons, they are vexations to the spirit.

If you compare yourself with others, you may become vain and bitter; for always there will be greater and lesser persons than yourself.

Enjoy your achievements as well as your plans.

Keep interested in your own career, however humble; it is a real possession in the changing fortunes of time.

Exercise caution in your business affairs; for the world is full of trickery.

But let this not blind you to what virtue there is; many persons strive for high ideals; and everywhere life is full of heroism.

Be yourself. Especially, do not feign affection.

Neither be cynical about love; for in the face of all aridity and disenchantment it is perennial as the grass.

Take kindly the counsel of the years, gracefully surrendering the things of youth.

Nurture strength of spirit to shield you in sudden misfortune.

But do not distress yourself with imaginings.

Many fears are born of fatigue and loneliness.

Beyond a wholesome discipline, be gentle with yourself.

You are a child of the Universe no less than the trees and the stars; you have a right to be here.

And whether or not it is clear to you, no doubt the Universe is unfolding as it should.

Therefore be at peace with God, whatever you conceive Him to be, and whatever your labors and aspirations, in the noisy confusion of life keep peace with your soul.

With all its sham, drudgery and broken dreams, it is still a beautiful world.

Be careful. Strive to be happy.

—Found in Old Saint Paul's Church, Baltimore. Dated 1692.

SEX

Sex and spirituality are very closely aligned. Sex can bring us to oneness with another human. It also has a potential Godlike power, the power of procreation. Sex is a powerful tool that can bring masculine and feminine and blend them as one. It can be the pinnacle of ultimate intimacy. On the other hand unhealthy sex can be the death of civilization. Just like any power or tool—like money it can be used for good or bad.

A healthy sexual relationship requires two whole and healthy individuals. It is essential that all the preceding chapters have been read and understood to maximize the opportunity of a healthy relationship thriving sexually. Communication is essential, we must be able to discuss our wants, needs and desires. It's not easy. Any worthwhile endeavor takes time, patience and perseverance.

The first step in healthy sexuality is getting in tune with your own sexual feelings and drives. Many of us were taught that sex is dirty. For many, sex was not discussed in the family. Some teenagers—feeling sexual drives either learned to repress them or feel guilty about them.

Many teenage boys hid in the bathroom and masturbated. Did these boys know that it was a normal and natural behavior? Do adult women and men realize that it's even not unusual for married men to masturbate on a weekly basis? How many women believe that they can become more in tune with their own sexual natures through self stimulation?

Once we accept our sexual natures, how do we express them? Sex is a wonderful gift that can give immense pleasure or cause tremendous sorrow. The difference lies in our development of values. That is why I saved this chapter for the last part of this section. For sex to be the rich fulfilling experience it is meant to be, there must be love and commitment. There needs to be honesty and communication between partners. Enough said, that's what this book is about.

What are the ingredients for delicious sex?

Food for Sex: The Way to Natural Love?

Since the beginning of time, it seems, men and women have been looking to foods to ignite their lover (or their own) sexual passion. It has been said, in fact and fiction that Casanova, Don Juan, Cleopatra, Aphrodite, and Marquis de Sade, known for their mysterious powers of seduction and amorous exploits, all relied on some form of aphrodisiac.

Around the world, various foods, herbs and rare, or extreme concoctions have been used as aphrodisiacs through the centuries, in hope that their special ingredients would somehow enhance a person's allure, increase fertility, improve vitality and sexual stamina.

Today, critics regard aphrodisiacs as quackery. Nevertheless, there is backing for at least some of the folk wisdom that has been passed down through the generations.

Chocolate—has long been reputed to be a food of love, its romantic reputation attributed to the fact that it is rich in the chemical phenylethylamine. According to psychiatrist Michael Liebowitz, M.D., author of *Chemistry of Love* (Little, Brown and Co.), the level of "some sort of amphetamine-like chemical in the brain, possibly phenylethylamine, goes up when we meet the right person." Chocolate also contains a small amount of caffeine, which stimulates the release and action of epinephrine, one of the neurotransmitters that triggers sexual arousal. The sugar added to chocolate offers a quick form of energy. Together, these ingredients may enhance arousal in some people.

Carrots—another food hailed as an aphrodisiac, is rich in beta-carotene, a nutrient that helps bolster sperm count and increase levels of important sex hormones.

Niacin—which improves circulation to sexual organs (and all parts of the body) is found in asparagus and figs. Figs are also rich in **Magnesium**—a mineral required to produce sex hormones. Apricots are another excellent source of magnesium (and beta-carotene).

Ginseng root—(Chinese, Korean & Russian) has been found to increase stamina and potency, without any harmful side-effects (other than a possible increase in blood-pressure).

Oysters—which have long been dubbed to have a positive effect on human sexuality, are rich in Zinc, which has been associated with an increase in sperm motility, which theoretically increases a man's fertility. It also helps reduce the risk of inflammation of the prostate,[59] a problem that can put a crimp in any man's love life.

Vitamin C—Scientific studies have found that 200 mg of vitamin C can detox sperm made sluggish by smoking and other pollutants, and Jean Carper, author of *Food-Your Miracle Medicine* (Harper-Collins) recommends 200-plus mg. doses in the form of any of these easy-to-eat foods (1 cantaloupe, 3 oranges, 2 1/2 cups raw strawberries, 1 1/2 red peppers, 3 kiwi fruit). Food is always preferred over supplements due to its content of other sperm helpers such as the antioxidant glutathione, found in leafy greens and avocado.

In order to function properly, the nervous systems natural hormones and neurotransmitters (which control physical and emotional arousal and excitement) require vitamins C and B-6, as well as amino acids which come from protein. Other necessary nutrients can be derived from such foods as whole grains, nuts &

---

[59] Prostatitis can be relieved with saw palmetto, flaxseed and a vegetarian diet.

seeds, legumes and green vegetables. Clearly, these foods provide nutrients that are helpful for sex.

A short list of edibles reputed to be aphrodisiacs might include artichokes, bamboo shoots, basil, caviar, game birds, garlic, grapes, halibut, horseradish, mackerel, leeks, mugwort, nutmeg, paprika, radishes, rosemary, saffron, sage and spinach.

Sometimes, these remedies work because the user believes they will or because they provide a vitamin or trace mineral the person lacks. *People don't feel sexy if they are unhealthy.*

Tips to Boost your Sexual Health

- **Eat a balanced diet**—including an abundance of healthy fruits and vegetables.

- **Use alcohol in moderation**—Excessive use suppresses sensation and decreases nerve response needed for arousal.

- **Don't smoke**—Nicotine increases the chance of infertility in women and impotence in men.

- **Exercise**—Study after study has shown that people who exercise on a regular basis had more libido than their less active counterparts.

- **Check medications**—Some may cause side effects that adversely affect sexual activity. Consult your physician or pharmacist, since the product label is unlikely to offer this information.

- **Stay away from drugs**—and the so-called over-the-counter sex enhances. Many are dangerous and actually impair performance.

- **Recommended supplements**—for sex are: Yohimbe, Ginkgo Biloba (see pg. 286), Damiana, Ginseng, Garlic, Zinc, niacin, vitamin B6, Arginine and everything recommended in the Reversing the Aging Process chapter.

Getting in the Mood

Mood itself is the ultimate aphrodisiac. Nothing can guarantee that you will "light someone's fire" unless you provide him, or her, with the proper atmosphere to spark the desire. Food and drink are only supplementary to the romantic task at hand, while the job of arousing interest in your partner does take two. Look for new ways to develop greater intimacy, self-confidence, and creativity, while reducing anxiety and guilt. Only a honest, sensitive approach and straight-forward communication can help.

I think sex is a good segue into the physical part of this book.

PHYSICAL HEALTH, CREATING THE PERFECT BODY

CREATING THE PERFECT BODY

12 Ways To Increase Your Metabolism

While millions of people starve to death in many parts of the world, the United States has the dubious honor of being the fattest country on the globe: Dieting is responsible for more than 400 deaths each year. Nearly 30 percent of adults and 26 percent of children are overweight or obese. And, according to two recent government surveys, the unhealthy numbers show no signs of lightening up: We're eating 231 more calories a day than we were 16 years ago, and the average weight of people aged 25 to 30 has increased by a whopping 10 pounds. In fact, one third more people are obese now than a decade ago. Although the extra pounds could be explained by exercise-induced muscle (which, inch for inch, weighs more than fat), it's not likely. The latest excuse for being fat is "the fat gene". **Well, our genes haven't changed over the last 20 years, however the way we fit into our jeans has changed.** *I will have more on this in the next chapter, Genetics and Obesity.* "The people in this country are still geared toward overeating," says Margaret McDowell, R.D., at the National Center for Health Statistics. If you don't want your over-eating to get the best of you, consider raising your basal metabolic rate.

Your basal metabolic rate is the rate at which your body utilizes energy while at rest. Put another way, it has to do with how efficiently your body burns calories. As you may recall from your physiology classes, calories are the measuring unit of heat energy. For the purposes of this chapter, when your metabolism is higher, you burn more fat and have an easier time losing weight (fat) or maintaining your ideal body weight.

Calculating your basal metabolic rate

Women	**Men**
weight X 4.3 = A	weight X 6.2 = A
height X 4.3 = B	height X 12.7 = B
A + B + 655 = C	A + B + 65 = C
age X 4.7 = D	age X 6.8 = D

$$C - D = BMR \text{ (Basal Metabolic Rate)}$$

This is the number of calories your body burns when it is resting. Your BMR may be higher or lower than what you have calculated. This chapter describes ways to increase your BMR.

Statistics reveal that most people are not happy with their weight or the shape of their body. Chances are you fit into this category. Half of the women and a fourth of the men in this country are currently trying to lose weight and reshape their bodies. A sad fact is that a majority of these people are going about it in the wrong way, like swimming upstream. Most people try and loose weight by dieting which usually involves eating certain foods and cutting back on calories.

Diets Don't Work!

Two out of three people who go on a diet will re-gain the weight in 1 year or less and 97% will re-gain the weight in 5 years. To make matters worse, a majority of dieters who loose weight will gain back **even more fat** than they had before they started the diet. They have violated the most important rule in creating and maintaining a healthy, fast metabolism; they lost lean body mass or muscle. Breaking this first rule is the reason most people get fatter as they age. Decreased activity leads to muscle loss. Why is lean muscle tissue so important?

1. *Muscle burns fat*—Muscle is a highly metabolic tissue; it burns five times as many calories as most other body tissues pound for pound. **The addition of 10 pounds of muscle to your body can burn 600 calories per day.** You would have to run 6 miles a day, seven days a week to burn the same number of calories. **Ten extra pounds of muscle can burn a pound of fat in one week**, that's 52 pounds of fat a year.

The best way to increase lean muscle mass is through resistance training which means weight lifting. A regular weight training program involving only 30 minutes, 3 times a week for about six months adds 10 pounds of muscle.[a] Isn't that fantastic? The wonderful news about increasing your metabolism through increasing your muscle mass is that **you don't have to restrict your calorie intake.**

2. *Grazing decreases fat storage*—The second way to increase your metabolism is to eat several small meals a day. This keeps your metabolism stoked. The typical dieter will often skip meals and, as research points out, **the worst meal to skip, if you want to increase your metabolism, is <u>breakfast</u>.** This temporary fasting state sends a signal to the body that food is scarce. As a result, the stress hormones (including cortisone) increase and the body begins "lightening the load" and shedding its muscle tissue. Decreasing this metabolically active tissue will decrease the body's need for food. By the next feeding, the pancreas is sensitized and will sharply increase blood insulin levels which is the body's signal to make fat. **Grazing (eating small meals every 2-3 hours) will decrease cholesterol 15%, decrease cortisol 17%, and decrease insulin 28%.**[b] Eating in this way will virtually prevent carbohydrates and proteins from being converted into fat. Have you ever wondered how the Sumo wrestlers get so big; they fast, and then gorge themselves with food.

---

[a] See the chapter: Exercise, to design your program.
[b] *Eat More, Weigh Less,* Dr. Dean Ornish.

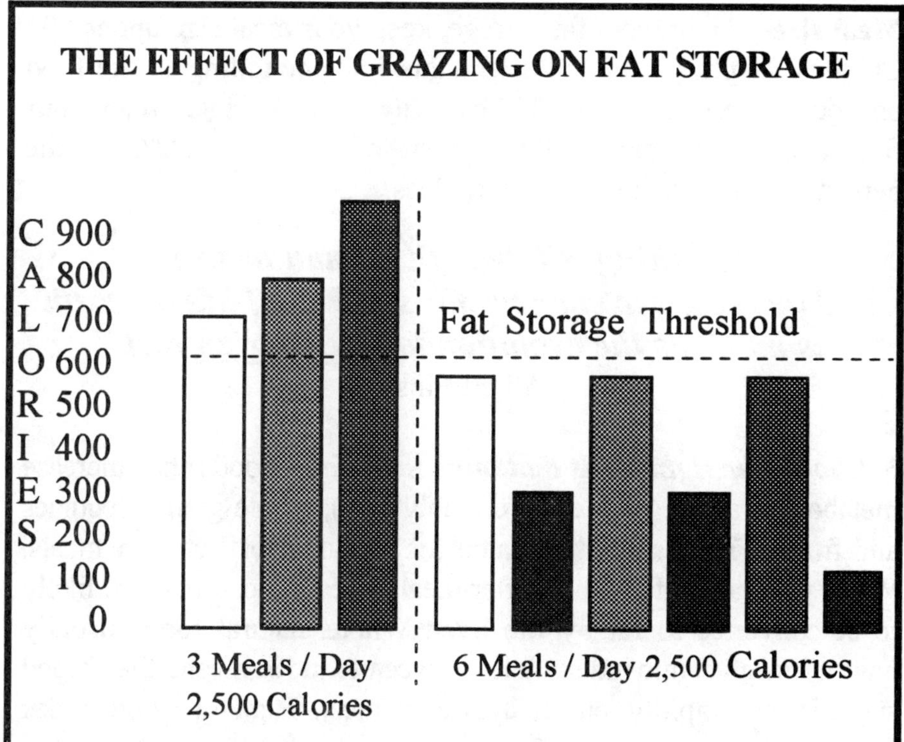

Fig. 1 This graph illustrates how 700 Calories can be stored as fat by eating three meals. No calories stored as fat by eating six meals, the same Calories.

Three meals a day

Breakfast of 700 Calories is 100 over the threshold
Lunch of 800 Calories is 200 over the threshold
Dinner of 1,000 Calories is 400 over the threshold
100 + 200 + 400 = 700 Calories stored as fat

Six meals a day

Three meals at 600 Calories plus two at 300 and one at 100 with none over the fat storing threshold produces no fat storage.

Meal size—To prevent fat storage, keep your meal size under 600 Calories. To physically understand this, imagine rolling all the food on your plate into a ball. This ball should be no bigger than your fist. This is assuming a fat content of less than 30%. If the percentage of fat is higher, then eat less.

> *"Nothing will benefit human health*
> *and increase the chances for survival of life on earth*
> *as much as the evolution to a vegetarian diet."*
> —Albert Einstein

3. *Choose the right foods that burn more fat*—Foods that increase metabolism are vegetables (preferably raw), whole grains, legumes and fruits. Fruits should be eaten for breakfast or between meals. When you eat fruits with or after meals, the fructose is more likely to be converted to fat by the liver. Whole, natural foods usually have a low glycemic index. A low glycemic index means that blood sugar is not rapidly elevated after a meal. High glycemic index foods, such as sugary foods, put your blood sugar on a rollercoaster. When blood sugar rises too rapidly, insulin is secreted in an overabundance. This excess insulin stimulates fat production and storage. The superfluous insulin will cause too much sugar to be stored resulting in low blood sugar. Low blood sugar, in turn, will then cause stress hormone release, depression, fatigue and hunger.

The high fiber in the recommended plant-based diet will actually slow digestion and absorption for a more even blood sugar level. Fiber will also bind with some fat and prevent its absorption. High fiber foods are beneficial for speeding up bowel transit time, too. This will take some stress off the liver as less toxins will form. The body can then more efficiently metabolize fats.

Foods that slow metabolism are sugars and fats. Fats not only have twice the calories, gram for gram, as carbohydrates and proteins, they also use only 2% of their calories to be stored as fat. Protein and carbohydrates, however, will burn about 25% of their calories to be stored as fat. For example, if you eat 3,000 calories a day and decrease the percentage of fat from 40% to 20%, then you can loose 1 pound of fat in about 3 weeks—while at the same time eating 20% more food from carbohydrates and protein. The bottom line is **EATING FAT MAKES YOU FAT!**

For those of you who drink alcohol, listen up. One of the greatest ways to sabotage fat loss is alcohol consumption. Aside from having 7 calories per gram, alcohol will shift metabolism in favor of fat deposition, burdening the liver and stimulating your appetite.

4. *Fight fat with fat*[c]—Sounds paradoxical, doesn't it? **Not all fats make you fat,** unless you eat too much. Omega-3 fatty acids can actually increase your metabolic rate. They also rid the body of excess fluids and can increase your energy level. The best source of Omega-3 fatty acids is from fresh organic flax seed or oil available in health foods stores;[d] deep sea fish is another source. Omega-6 fatty acids (especially gamma linolenic acid or GLA) are also essential to health and a healthy metabolism but are less likely to be deficient in a healthy diet. Good sources of GLA and Omega-6 fatty acids are borage seed oil, black current oil and primrose oil.

5. *Supplements can increase fat metabolism*[e]—Good nutrition is extremely important in maintaining and boosting your metabolism The best nutrition comes from whole foods such as whole grains, vegetables, legumes (beans, peas and lentils) and fruits. If you eat processed, non-organic foods, if you lead a stressful life or live in a polluted environment, then it would behoove you to include some supplements that have a positive effect on your metabolism. Superfoods such as algaes[f], wheat and barley grasses, and kelp can

---

[c] See the chapter: Deadly Fats vs. Healing Fats.
[d] Good sources: Omega Fortified Flax or
Organic Flax Seed Oil made by Spectrum Naturals
[e] See the chapter: Why Supplements?
[f] Including spirulina, chlorella and blue-green algae.

add special nutrients not always found in a healthy diet or other supplements. The plethora of vitamins, minerals and essential fatty acids will increase the efficiency of oxidation and raise metabolic rate, energy and activity level. The protein in these superfoods can increase metabolism 30% compared to 10% of a purely carbohydrate meal. Protein will also decrease fatigue often experienced after a low protein lunch or other meal.

Percentage of Calories from Protein	
Most fruits	5-8%
Whole grains	10-20%
Legumes	25-30%
Most vegetables	30-50%
Mori-Nu Tofu "Lite"	>60%

Proteins are made of amino acids one amino acid that is very important in fat metabolism is carnitine. Carnitine actually carries fatty acids into the cell's "furnace" or mitochondria. Carnitine is especially helpful for vegetarians who may not be getting enough methionine and lysine (carnitine is made from these two amino acids). Taking a gram of carnitine a day can prevent a deficiency.

If your diet is like most Americans, the **SAD** diet (Standard American Diet), you are likely deficient in chromium and should supplement with about 400 mcg per day. This will help your body loose more fat and retain muscle tissue.

In the chapter Reversing The Aging Process, I discuss the marvelous benefits of CoQ-10, DHEA and other supplements that help with fat burning.

Another popular weight loss supplement is Citrimax, this is an appetite supressant that temporarily blocks the conversion of carbohydrates into fat.

6. *Some herbs can stoke your metabolic fire.* Herbal combinations are currently very popular for increasing thermogenesis. The three main herbs used in a variety of formulas are mahuang (ephedra), guarana or kola nut and white willow bark. Ephedra contains ephedrine; guarana and kola nut contain caffeine; white willow bark contain salicylate like aspirin. These three, in the right proportions, have been shown to increase thermogenesis (heat production) and burn calories. Anyone with high blood pressure, heart problems or other medical problems should consult with their physician before taking these herbs.

Other herbs serve as adaptogens to balance the body's homeostatic systems and help you adapt to stress. These include ginseng (Siberian and Korean), astragulus, gotu kola, schizandra and licorice root.

7. *Spices can burn calories and decrease sugar cravings.* Some of the spices that increase metabolism are ginger, cayenne pepper and mustard. For example, dry mustard can increase metabolism percent for up to 3 hours with less than 1 teaspoon. In a British study, eating 3/5 teaspoon hot pepper sauce raised the metabolism 25 percent, burning an extra 45 calories in three hours. In an Australian animal test, ginger increased the metabolism 20 percent. The spices that help control blood sugar and sugar cravings are cinnamon, clove and bay leaf. (Note: The minerals chromium and vanadium also help control blood sugar levels and sugar cravings.) Spices and herbs can stimulate the potency of insulin so you require less of the hormone to process sugar, says Richard Anderson of the U.S. Department of Agriculture. This could be very important for people with Type II diabetes. Anderson's tests found sage and oregano double insulin activity; turmeric and cloves triple the activity; cinnamon is most potent, Dose: amounts common in foods. Cinnamon also may lower blood pressure, according to new research at George Washington University.

153

8. *Water washes away fat.* Water is very important in helping to maintain a healthy metabolic rate. Three quarts a day, between meals, is optimum. In fact, water may be the most important catalyst to increase fat burning. Water suppresses your appetite naturally.

High water intake will reduce fat deposits by taking a load off the liver. The liver's main functions are detoxification and metabolism. The kidneys can get rid of toxins and spare the liver if they have sufficient water. This allows the liver to metabolize more fat. Adequate water will also decrease bloating and edema caused by fluid accumulation. Water does this by flushing out sodium and toxins. A high water intake also helps relieve constipation by keeping your stools soft. Simply DRINKING ONE GALLON OF WATER throughout the day, that's cooled to 40 degrees, WILL BURN 300 CALORIES, the equivalent of running three miles.

9. *Moderate doses of sunlight increase metabolism.* The sun has been getting alot of bad press lately. Actually, sunlight in moderation is very good for the body in a variety of ways, including increasing your metabolism as documented in the excellent book, *Sunlight*, by Zane Kime, M.D. (World Health Publications, 1980) in it he writes, "There is conclusive evidence that exposure to sunlight produces a metabolic effect in the body very similar to that produced by physical training, and is definitely followed by a measured improvement in physical fitness." He also explains in this book how a vegan (no dairy or egg vegetarian diet) diet will greatly decrease the risk of skin cancer.

10. *Saunas can burn hundreds of calories in minutes.* Dry saunas will give your body an aerobic workout with the cooler infrared saunas burning up to 900 calories in one 30 minute session, according to research. A typical hot air dry sauna will burn approximately 300 calories in 30 minutes at a temperature of 180-235 degrees F. An infrared sauna, on the other hand, will burn approximately 900 calories in the same 30 minutes at only 110-130 degrees. Infrared energy is used to keep premature babies warm so it is perfectly safe. The reason this low temperature, comfortable sauna burns more than three times as many calories as a conventional dry sauna has to do with its deep heat penetration. It invokes two to three times the sweat volume of a hot air sauna. One gram of sweat requires the body to burn 0.586 Kcal. Like aerobic exercise, your metabolism remains higher for hours after an infrared sauna.

11. *Aerobic exercise can increase or decrease metabolism.* The best exercise for permanent fat loss is resistance training (lifting weights) because it increases muscle which burns more calories. Low intensity aerobic exercise such as walking is also an excellent way to burn fat efficiently. Furthermore, it will even increase your metabolic rate for hours after exercising. According to Dean Ornish, M.D., in his book *Eat More, Weigh Less*, intense exercise (beyond your target heart rate) may actually decrease your metabolism in the long run because you burn valuable muscle tissue.

In a study, Dr. John Duncan took 102 sedentary women and divided them into three groups. Each group walked three miles, five days a week for six months. The first group walked 5 mph, the second group 4 mph, and the third group 3 mph. He found that the slowest walking group lost the most weight. Running, or any aerobic exercise that raises heart rate above 80% of maximum (220-age x 0.8) will cause you to burn more muscle and less fat. An exercise heart rate kept closer to 60% of maximum (220-age x 0.6) or 108 beats per minute for a 40 year old person, will burn mostly fat. This is why walking is superior to running as a fat burning exercise. Perhaps the worst problem with excessive exercise is the dropout level. More people will burnout and quit exercise altogether if they overdo it.

12. ***The time of day you exercise can affect your metabolism.*** It has been found that the best time to exercise is before a meal simply because exercise suppresses appetite and increases metabolism. If you are interested in losing weight and increasing your metabolism, walk before a meal.

Diets or calorie restriction doesn't work in the long run. Increase your metabolism instead and you'll feel and look better while taking control of your weight.

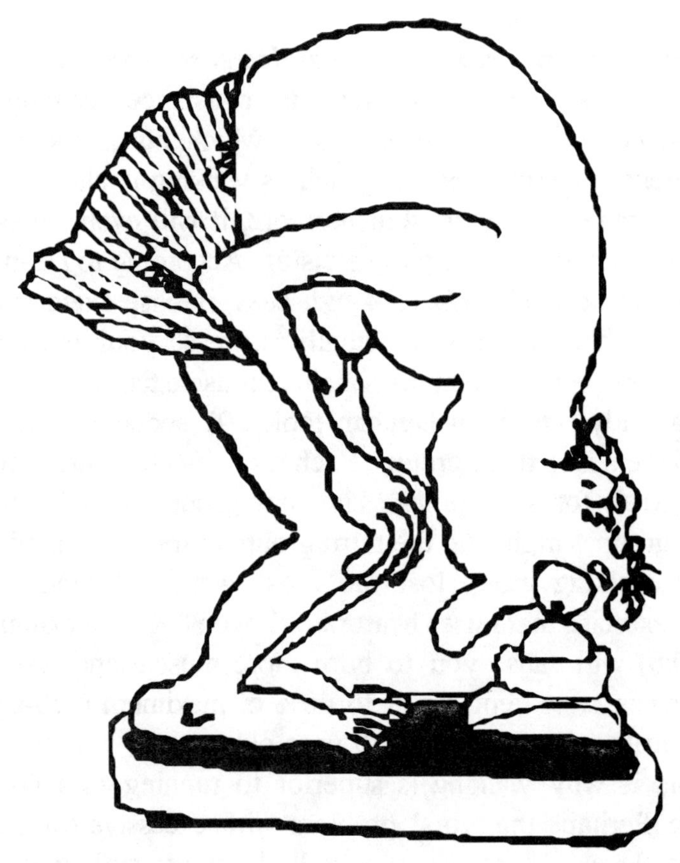

GENETICS AND OBESITY

Jenny eats plenty, about 3,000 Calories a day for her 135 pound body, but only 60 grams of fat, which are 18% of her total calories. Susie tries to stick to 2,000 calories, but she eats the typical Standard American Diet **(SAD)** with about 40% of calories from fat. This is 90 grams of fat, more than she burns most days, so she stores surplus fat.

Many individuals, like Susie think they have a genetic tendency to become overweight. This belief was reinforced by a report in 1994 that a gene in mice could malfunction and cause obesity, and that there may be a parallel process in humans.

That report has given overweight people an excuse to be obese. They now believe they are victims of their genetics.

The study found a gene in mice that causes fat cells to produce a protein that signals when the body has enough fat. This protein tells the body when to quit storing fat. If the gene malfunctions the signal protein is not made, and fat continues to be stored.

This is easy to understand given plenty of fat. Suppose the fat supply is limited—in other words, consider a low-fat diet. If extra fat is not there it can't be stored, so this genetic extrapolation from mice to men shouldn't cause a problem. Right?

Some might argue that if the defective gene doesn't tell the body to quit storing fat and there is no more available in the diet, then the body will say "I've gotta have more fat so I'll make the darned stuff." We're back to the old conversion of carbohydrate to fat story. The question of what is more important Calorie counting (total calorie balance) or restricting fat intake to just what you need (fat balance).

If you're like Susie and believe the amount of food you eat is the main factor in controlling your weight, and your genes will decide if you'll turn it into fat, look at the research.

There is a large record of studies on the dietary fate of carbohydrate that go back more than 30 years. This includes biochemical studies, clinical studies on animals and people, and epidemiological studies. The largest proportion of these data can be explained if the principal source of stored body fat is eating excess fat. Under normal dietary and metabolic conditions, the conversion of carbohydrate to fat is negligible (less than 2%, according to the numbers). When dietary fat is restricted to less than is needed to meet the needs for essential body fats, then your body can manufacture fat from carbohydrate, but only if you over-eat massive amounts of carbohydrate.

A study that found significant conversion of carbohydrate to fat and weight gain, fed people 3,500 to 5,000 calories, restricted their fat intake to 3%, and did not let the group exercise. Note, that not only did it take massive over-feeding to stimulate fat production from carbohydrate, it took severe fat restriction.

If you starve your body of fat and pig out on too many calories (large meals), then the surplus is converted to fat and stored.

Overall, the evidence that eating too much fat is the main cause of excess stored body fat is large and convincing. Those who disagree ignore the majority of the data and rely on a few studies that are ambiguous. They are also big on anecdotal stories of weight gain on low-fat diets. The unanswered question is whether these stories are not really about low-fat diets, but fat starvation diets, in which case they are consistent with the clinical nutrition data.

The message is eat low-fat, not no fat. Eric Jequier, Ph.D., at the University of Lausanne, Switzerland, wrote in a recent review of published studies "Fat synthesis from carbohydrate in adipose tissue is of little importance." This means that when you eat a balanced low-fat diet, you won't manufacture fat. So far there have been five studies of low-fat (20% to 25% of total calories), unrestricted-calorie diets for overweight people: in each case, they lost weight.

You are more likely to gain weight easily if your parents are overweight. Doesn't this emphasize that there is a strong genetic component? Yes, in some cases, but perhaps not as often as we tend to believe. The difficulty with family studies on overweight people is that it's hard to separate genetic effects from learned habits.

Overweight parents who eat too much fat tend to provide the same food choices for their children as for themselves, so their kids eat too much fat, too. This is not genetics; this is eating what is available.

Fortunately, at an early age children have an instinct for high levels of physical activity—they play a lot. Unfortunately, this doesn't last too long, and surely the emergence of overweight children grows out of a continued consumption of fat coupled with a gradual slide in the level of physical activity.

There are studies on identical twins that suggest when they are brought up in different environments, if one is obese it is probable that the other will be too.

The estimates of experts in the field, such as Claude Bouchard, Ph.D., at Laval University in Quebec, are that the heritability of obesity in twins may be as high as 70%. In the general population it is closer to 20% to 25%, although it can be as high as 40%. These estimates say that although a significant amount of obesity is connected with genetics, a larger amount is not.

There is another troubling aspect of the genetic link. Data shows that Americans have the highest incidence of obesity in developed countries; for example, obesity is twice as prevalent in the U.S. as in France (small wonder our heart disease rate is so much higher; you don't need the Mediterranean diet to explain this).

The U.S. is a nation of immigrants. Do we really believe our current rate of obesity has become so much higher than people in the countries of Europe, Asia, and Africa from whom we descend, by genetic changes in so few generations? This does not seem reasonable. Besides, Asians who emigrate to the U.S. and change to American eating habits tend to become more overweight than those

159

who stay home. Weight gain does not wait for genetics, it crops up in a single generation and therefore is due mainly to the **SAD** diet, aided by less physical activity. The average American weighs ten pounds more today than they did less than twenty years ago. Nearly one third of Americans have become obese. Our genetics haven't changed in this short time, fat consumption and activity level has. There is a genetic influence that can be explained by the body types we inherit.

Body types

There are three body types 1.) ectomorph (small body frame), 2.) mesomorph (medium body frame) and 3.) endomorph (large body frame). Through helping people to get in shape I have observed that ectomorphs tend to be slender they need to eat more healthy fat and protein to gain lean body mass. Mesomorphs only need to exercise and eat right. Endomorphs are genetically programmed to be big, the choice is to be muscular or fat. Endomorphs want to eat more calories, they feel deprived when they don't get them. Endomorphs have the most difficulty with fat. They absolutely need to put on muscle and restrict their fat intake. If you are this type, you need to follow the recommendations for increasing your metabolism and definitely increase your muscle mass.

If your parents are overweight it is important not to be complacent, shrug, and say "I can't fight family history."

Many diet studies use self-report data, which are notoriously unreliable; sometimes people under-reported their food intake by as much as 100%. Many obese people tend to over eat, snacking on such high fat foods as chips, doughnuts, and candy. **We have**

not seen published reports of obese people who compulsively over-eat on fruits and vegetables: FAT IS THE PROBLEM.

What is more, in many overweight people there is a large psychological factor, and it is immeasurably hard for them to change their eating habits. There is plenty of evidence that suggests this could help because there are obese people who achieve weight control through diet and exercise when they persevere.

In summary, to put the study on obese mice into perspective, genetics may be one of the important factors in overweight problems. This should not get in the way of recognizing the main cause of being overweight is eating too much fat coupled with too little physical activity. Rather than waiting expectantly for the next magic potion, genetic engineering, which may help some people with weight control problems, we need to hammer at the same old message: limit your fat intake:

> **Convert your desired body weight to kilograms by multiplying pounds by 0.454 (or dividing by 2.2). This is the average number of grams of fat per day you may eat.**

To lose body fat, this number should be reduced by up to one half keeping in mind that healthy fat is essential to good health.[g]

There has been some recent evidence from the Calorie lab that some people burn fat more slowly than others do, however, the bottom line of their research showed that **fat restriction coupled with exercise always resulted in fat loss** as long as this lifestyle change was maintained. In my years of practice as a physician and a fitness trainer, I learned how to get different types of people in shape and keep them in shape. Metabolism of fat seems to be different in every individual. Most highly active people can eat 30% of their calories from healthy fat[h] while most sedentary individuals need to decrease their fat intake to below 20% and get

---

[g] See the chapter: Deadly Fats vs. Healing Fats.
[h] See the chapter: Deadly Fats vs. Healing Fats.

more active. Unfortunately, **fat tends to anesthetize the brain** and produce lethargy. This makes it difficult to get started. Another road block is the difficulty in radically changing from the SAD diet that is high in fat, sugar and salt, because the body will desperately crave these substances when they are denied. In my past dietary foibles, I noticed that if I ate salty foods in a few hours I would crave sugary foods and vice-versa. It takes about three weeks to break the habit and learn to enjoy healthy foods. The positive aspect of this is, if you persist and go three weeks with just healthy foods you will actually enjoy them. Your taste buds will be rejuvenated and you will experience subtle tastes like never before.

My challenge to you is to make a commitment for just three weeks. The reason for three weeks is that 21 days is the period of time it takes to break a bad habit and establish a new one. It won't be easy, but I guarantee it will be worth it.

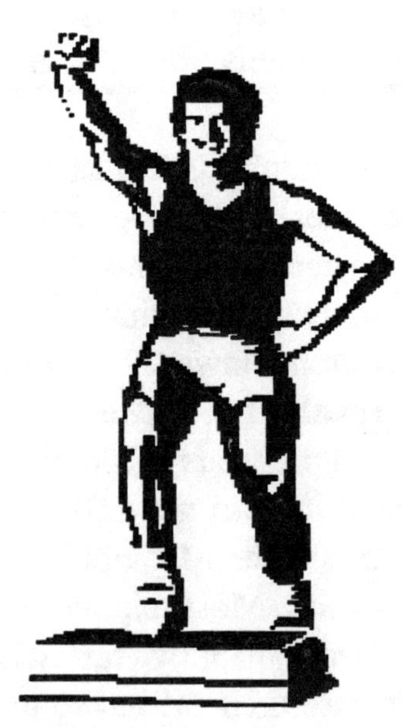

HEALING POWER OF TOUCH

The healing power of touch has been known thoughout history. Today, we recognize its physical, emotional and spiritual healing qualities. While in medical school I learned that patients who were touched by nurses and doctors healed faster, infants would die without touch and that the more touch babies received the healthier they became. Dr. Saul Schanberg of Duke University found that because vision is blurred and hearing is not well developed, touch is "possibly the most critical of all senses to the newborn." A study of 40 premature babies was done by Dr. Schanberg and Dr. Tiffany Field of the University of Miami. Half of the babies selected at random were gently stroked for 45 minutes a day. The other 20 were not. Although fed the same amount of calories ten days later the touched babies were 47 percent heavier, more alert and more socially responsive than the unstimulated group. Don't worry, touch won't make you gain weight unless you are significantly under weight.

Recently, their studies have shown massage of premature babies can save 4 billion dollars each year; the money is saved in a shorter hospital stay. Field also found that massage stokes the immune system. In one study by colleague Gail Ironson, M.D., HIV-positive men were given 45-minute massages, five days a week, for a month. "They showed an increase in serotonin," Field says, "and an increase in natural killer cells, the first line of defense in the immune system." Children and adolescents hospitalized for psychiatric problems displayed remarkable reductions in anxiety levels and positive attitude changes. Massage made preschoolers more focused, and adult office-workers more alert. **Massage improves immune function and significantly reduces anxiety and stress.**

Researchers have found that when rats lick their young, it stimulates the production of growth hormones in the infants. Rats had less brain cell deterioration and memory loss if handled 15 minutes a day during the first three weeks of life. The necessity of touch is seen throughout the animal kingdom but, it seems to be especially important to mammals. All mammals nurse their young and touch doesn't end there. Watch a documentary on primates, you will see how apes, baboons and other primates use touch. Think about how pets respond to touch—kittens purr and dogs will do close to anything for touch, the more the better. Petting animals doesn't just benefit the animal, it seems to convey the same benefits to the one doing the petting—karma!, The health benefits of pets is a chapter in itself. My recommendation is for anyone that needs more touch in their life go to the pound and rescue an animal.

Experiment gone wrong !

Studies on rabbits fed high cholesterol diets gave mixed results. When thoroughly investigated it was discovered that the rabbits in the lower, reachable cages were petted and the rabbits in higher cages weren't. The result was petted rabbits had 60% less artery blockage than the unpetted.

In 1987, five Atlanta nurses began the National Association for Nurse Massage Therapists (NANMT) which had grown to about 500 members by the end of 1993. These nurses report that patients receiving massages take fewer narcotics, hypnotics and sedatives for pain and sleeplessness, than those not receiving massages It also helps patients cope with hospital stress. Massage creates a relaxation response which results in decreased heart rate, blood pressure and skin temperature. **Massage enhances healing physiologically, psychologically, neurologically and spiritually.**

Michael I. Weintraub, M.D., clinical professor of neurology at New York Medical College, conducted an experiment, treating 63 patients with a twice-weekly regimen of massage and Shiatsu acupressure for four weeks. Half had not responded to other remedies, but 86 percent of them showed decreased pain and increased mobility by the fifth session. Weintraub now has several massage therapists working in his office. "After one month of therapy, we can judge whether people can return to work, and how permanent their symptoms are," says Weintraub, noting that it takes three to six months of physical therapy to reach the same point. In my own practice, I always begin and end a visit with a touch. When it feels appropriate I exchange hugs.

In the book *Hands-on Healing,* Rodale Press, there are descriptions of over thirty types of hands-on healing. Most of these include massage.

Acupressure, Reflexology, Zone Therapy and Shiatsu rely on the use of pressure points to balance spiritual energy. These points are located along different meridians on the body. Each point represents a different organ or areas of the body. Trager and Polarity Therapy use rocking and shaking movements. Despite all the methods from all over the world, it is touch that does the healing. I prefer a good old fashion massage for its health benefits. Others may prefer different methods. While, the healing qualities of massage are manifest in body, mind and spirit, the physical benefits are the easiest to notice.

Physical benefits of massage—Massage exerts its numerous healing effects through many systems—circulatory, neurological, endocrine and musculo-skeletal.

Massage helps circulation in three ways; it increases blood flow, it boosts the oxygen carrying capacity of blood up to 15% and it increases lymphatic circulation. Lymph is a milky white fluid filled with wastes from our cell's metabolic reactions and fluid that capillaries left behind. Lymph glands are located throughout the lymphatic system, they play an essential role in protecting us from disease and infection. The lymph does not circulate as the blood does, it has its own system that returns fluids. Lymphatic drainage depends largely on the squeezing effect of muscular contractions or massage.[i] It is easy to see how muscular activity is essential to our health. Massage can help loosen contracted, shortened muscles and can stimulate weak, flaccid muscles. This muscle balancing can help posture and can provide for more efficient movement. Massage does not increase muscle strength, but it can promote recovery from the fatigue that occurs after exercise.

Massage stimulates metabolism by stimulating and soothing the nervous system and aids in the excretion of wastes partly by increasing the body's secretions and excretions. It helps the skin to become softer and more supple.

Psychological effects—We all have stress in our daily lives relating to work, family, environment, society. Stress can make us sick both physically and emotionally. Mental tensions, frustrations, and insecurity are among the most damaging. Stress causes the release of hormones that create vasoconstriction (vessel shrinking) resulting in reduced circulation. Stress causes the heart to work harder, breathing to become rapid and shallow, and digestion to slow. Every body process is degraded by stress. Psychosomatic studies show how stress factors can cause migraines, peptic ulcers, hypertension, depression, etc. Soothing and relaxing massage can help by counteracting stress effects.

Dr. Hans Selye, in his book *The Stress of Life*, writes that too much stress for too long can be very harmful. These days, most people are aware that the chronic condition of stress in which the renowned "type A" personality lives (the person who constantly pushes himself or herself to achieve and produce) leads to heart attack and poor cardiovascular health. In fact, many researchers and health professionals are now saying that chronic stress can be considered the underlying cause of most diseases.

---

[i] In a disease of the lymphatic system—elephantiasis, legs and arms can swell to elephant like proportions—hence the name elephantiasis.

Here's what Selye says about the two major ways that stress can profoundly affect our health and well-being.

1. By activating the "fight or flight mechanism" of the sympathetic nervous system, stress takes blood away from our digestive tract and sends it to our muscles, readying us for action. this is why chronic stress usually harms our digestion and assimilation first—and then weakened digestion and assimilation over a period of time can lead to immune deficiencies resulting in cancer, chronic viral infections and a host of other diseases. It can also lead to a fundamental reduction in our vitality.

2. By reducing blood circulation to vital organs such as the brain, kidneys and liver, chronic stress deprives these organs of vital nutrients such as oxygen, sugars, vitamins and other substances that aid in repair of damaged tissues.

Massage has a definite psychological effect. Since massage animates the tactile sense, the body's primary sense, it brings people into the here and now and away from tension generated by constant preoccupation with problems. Also, loosening of muscle tension or armoring can lead to freeing of repressed emotions.

Users of massage as a healing tool realize quickly that they have found a form of drugless therapy. Headaches, insomnia, constipation, and minor aches and pains often respond. Massage can have a spectacular effect on nervous people who have been dependent on their pharmacy for rest and relaxation.

> National Institute of Health, N.I.H.
> has recently reported an 86% success rate
> in treating chronic low back pain with
> massage.

The theories of massage are scientific in character, but the actual use of these theories is an art, it involves the healing sense, sensitivity of touch and intuition. I believe there is a real power to the "laying on of hands" there are many methods of healing that aren't massage, which involve touch. There are some methods that only require spiritual touch, such as spiritual energy balancing.[j]

More Closeness and Intimacy—Another benefit of massage is increased intimacy and emotional connection. It is not unusual for some one to begin crying when being hugged or massaged. Touch by another sensitive caring individual can release trapped emotions. Most of us don't receive enough non-sexual touch.

Dr. Barbara DeAngelis, world renown relationship expert and author of several best-selling books including, *Are You the One For Me?* feels that massage is a terrific way to foster closeness and intimacy. She maintains, "one of the biggest problems between couples is the lack of real intimacy. In my workshops, I teach people that every moment is an opportunity to make love, whether we express that love sexually or not. I suggest scheduling what I call 'planned intimacy;' time when you plan to be together with someone you feel close with, without specifically planning to be sexually intimate. This is a perfect time to give and receive a massage with your partner." She explains that massage is an ideal way to express one's love and caring for another person through the hands. To be touched lovingly, without feeling like someone is trying to "turn you on" can create a great deal of trust and intimacy between two people. She adds that one of women's common complaints about loving relationships is that they don't get enough non-sexual touching and caressing. Massage is not only a wonderful way to receive that nurturing touch, but also a way to teach your partner how you would like them to touch you.

---

[j] See the chapter: chakras.

HUGGING

"We need 4 hugs a day for survival.
We need 8 hugs a day for maintenance.
We need 12 hugs a day for growth."
—Virginia Satir

Hugging is healthy. It helps the body's immune system, it keeps you healthier, it cures depression, it reduces stress, it induces sleep, it's invigorating, it's rejuvenating, it has no unpleasant side effects. Hugging is nothing less than a miracle drug.

Hugging is all natural. It is organic, naturally sweet, no pesticides, no preservatives, no artificial ingredients and 100 percent wholesome.

Hugging is practically perfect. There are no movable parts, no batteries to wear out, no periodic check-ups, low energy consumption, high energy yield, inflation proof, non-fattening, no monthly payments, no insurance requirements, theft-proof, nontaxable, non-polluting and of course, fully returnable.

Author Unknown

Tools—It is best to massage with oil, so your hands can apply pressure and, at the same time, move smoothly over the surface of the skin. Oil fulfills this function better than anything else. Because skin will absorb much of the oil, so use a healthful oil, not petroleum products like baby oil or mineral oil. I personally use cold-pressed almond oil by *Spectrum Naturals* which is available in most health food stores. If you plan on making massage a regular part of your health program at home, buy a massage table. The price of portable tables run from as low as $250.00 for a 24" wide table with no head rest (face cradle) to about $650.00 for a wide table with good covering and a headrest. For most people, a headrest or similar attachment is preferable as it permits lying face down without twisting the neck and for people with neck tension and/or injuries, a headrest is essential.

Ambiance—Make the room as comfortable as possible, adjust the temperature to keep the recipient of the massage comfortable. Dim the lights, and play tranquil, soothing music,[k] Fill the room with a beautiful relaxing scent, lavender is one of my favorites.

Clothing is optional, I kept my underwear on my first time. Except for intimate friends, draping should be used to cover body areas not being massaged. Your recipient should feel safe, secure and comfortable at all times.

Technique—It is not important where you start. Personally, I think starting with the feet will relax the rest of the body—the back is also a good starting point. Work across the body or proceed up the same side. Make sure you have some methodical way of covering every part of the body that is to be massaged. When I massage someone for the first time I ask them which areas need work and which areas they consider too personal for touch. Inner thighs, butt, chest and abdominals may be too personal for the first massage. As trust develops, that may change. It is best to start the massage with the recipient face down, let the recipient choose.

Make sure you don't strain your muscles while giving a massage or you will need a massage yourself. While it is nice to trade massages, I am too relaxed after a massage to give one, I want to "bathe in the afterglow."

Your nails need to be trimmed as short as possible and filed smooth. Otherwise, acupressure becomes acupuncture! Wear cool loose clothing and keep your center of gravity over the areas you are working, to minimize the chance of back strain.

---

[k] I like music by Enya, Steven Halpern and David Ackerman.

Unless you are medically trained don't work on people of questionable health.

Begin with light massage, then determine how hard you can massage, always keep it a pleasant experience. Have your recipient let you know if you are pushing too hard or too soft. While the best massage is vigorous, pay attention to any increased muscle tenseness and lighten up. As you become more proficient, you will notice muscular knots. These are areas of pent up energy and releasing them will result in increased relaxation and balancing of energy—and of course healing. To release knots, begin with light pressure and slowly increase it as tolerated until the knot is gone.

Giving and receiving a massage is a wonderful experience, similar to the need for food and shelter. Make sure you get your share of touch—it will be a healing experience.

PETS

Pets are good for your health. Studies have shown that pet owners are healthier and happier than people without pets. In one study of 91 heart attack patients 28% of those without pets died within one year. Only 6% of the pet owners died. A study of 938 senior citizens was performed by a health maintenance organization. They found that pet owners had less office visits than those without pets.

J.A. Serpell of the University of Cambridge studied 71 adults who acquired pets from the local animal shelter. Serpell assessed the health of these new pet owners at one, six and ten months. Overall, the pet owners reported a 50% reduction in minor health problems and improvement in psychological well-being. The physical and psychological well-being lasted longer in the dog owners. This may be from the exercise of walking the dog. Paul Dudley White, M.D. once gave this advice for health & fitness:

> ***"Walk your dog every day,***
> ***whether you have a dog or not."***

Throughout my life I have had just about every kind of pet there is. They all have their positive qualities. Cats are cool. Rats and fish are easy to care for. Trust your intuition and pick one. I have found dogs are the most loving.

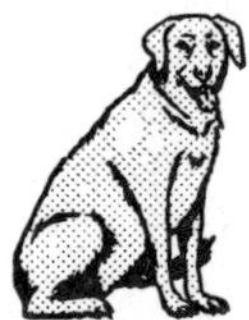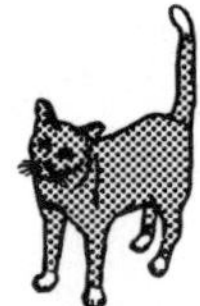

A Dog's Prayer

Treat me kindly, my beloved master for no heart in the world is more grateful for kindness than the loving heart of me.

Do not break my spirit with a stick, for though I lick your hand between the blows, your patience and understanding will more quickly teach me the things you would have me do.

Speak to me often, for your voice is the world's sweetest music, as you must know by the fierce wagging of my tail when your footstep falls upon my waiting ear.

When it is cold and wet, please take me inside, for I am now a domesticated animal, no longer used to bitter elements. And I ask no greater glory than the privilege of sitting at your feet beside the hearth. Though had you no home, I would rather follow you through ice and snow than rest upon the soft pillow in the warmest home in all the land, for you are my god and I am your devoted worshiper.

Keep my pan filled with fresh water, for although I should not reproach you were it dry, I cannot tell you when I suffer thirst.

Feed me clean food, that I may be well, to romp and play and do your bidding, to walk by your side, and stand ready, willing and able to protect you with my life should your life be in danger.

And, beloved master, should the Great Master see fit to deprive me of my health or sight, do not turn me away from you. Rather hold me gently in your arms as skilled hands grant me the merciful boon of eternal rest ... and I will leave you knowing with the last breath I drew, my fate was ever safest in your hands.

—Anonymous

PLANTS

If pets for any reason are not practical, then plants may be an option. Plants are very good for your health. They remove pollutants in the air and convert them to harmless substances better than any air filter. In 1973, NASA discovered that the air inside Skylab was contaminated with over 100 toxic chemicals. Development of air purification was essential to the future of space exploration. Thanks to the CIA, NASA learned that the Russians were experimenting with plants as air purifiers.

A research team was formed. They found that virtually all house plants suck pollutants into their leaves and destroy them—even the microorganisms in the soil neutralize toxins. My personal favorites are the peace lily and the spider plant. Both of these plants are hardy fighters of pollution. I bought a small peace lily three years ago for a couple dollars and now it is 4 ft. tall and 3 ft. wide. If I forget to water it, it starts to droop—if I water it, within a day or two it returns to perfect health—it is easy to care for. In addition to these, the most environmentally efficient (and easiest to maintain) are bamboo, areca and other palms, Boston fern, English Ivy, corn plants, chrysanthemums and philodendron. It takes about one medium sized plant for every 100 sq.ft. (10 ft by 10 ft room). The more plants, the cleaner the air.

SLEEP

Good quality sleep is as essential to our health as nutrition and exercise. It is while sleeping that our body does its healing. When we are deprived of sleep, we get sick. If we are sick, sleep is essential for healing.

How much sleep do we need? It depends on numerous factors: age, health, stress levels and genetics. Physically, we need more sleep when we are growing, maturing or healing. Psychologically and neurologically we need more sleep when we are learning or experiencing stress. The bottom line is body wisdom. If you need an alarm clock, and you still feel tired when it goes off—you are not getting the sleep **your** body needs.

Go to bed one hour earlier each week until you can wake up relaxed, refreshed and eager to face the day ahead. Remember, genetically we are programmed for a 25 hour day and it is not unusual to want to stay up an extra hour each night.

What do you do if you can't sleep?
1. Follow the dietary guidelines in this book.
2. Restrict the caffeine and alcohol in your diet.
3. Don't eat large meals 4 hours before bedtime.
4. Develop a ritual before bedtime eg. take a warm relaxing bath or shower, journal[l] then read this book until you are ready to sleep.
5. Reserve your bed and bedroom for sleeping and making love, not for TV or work.
6. Eat a piece of whole grain bread with fruit spread[m] 1 hr. before you plan to go to bed. This increases the serotonin in your brain. Serotonin is a neurotransmitter associated with a relaxed calm feeling.

---

[l] See the chapter Journaling.
[m] Or other small complex carbohydrate meal.

7. If needed, take melatonin and/or an herbal sleep formula with valerian, passion flower, skullcap and chamomile.
8. Don't count sheep, count your breaths: inhale, exhale 1, inhale, exhale 2, inhale, exhale 3, inhale, exhale 4, now start over. This will help to drive the thoughts from your mind that are keeping you awake. Sometimes you need to get up and write these thoughts down before you can sleep.

Sleep not only is good for our health, it saves lives and money. A study done by the (U.S.) National Commission on Sleep Disorders looked at the year, 1988. The cost of sleep-related accidents was $56 billion dollars in the U.S., the human cost was 25,000 lives and two-and-a-half million disabling injuries due to sleep-related accidents.

Stanford University did a study of its students, all of who were getting about seven-and-a-half hours of sleep, which is about average for their group, none of them had any complaints. The researchers asked them to sleep nine hours, an extra hour-and-a-half. They all complained bitterly, "We're not going to have time to study. It's going to ruin our social life." It turned out that when they did sleep nine hours, they not only felt better, but on the average their grades went up about 10 percent.

Dr. Stanley Coren of the University of British Columbia, psychologist and author of, *Sleep Thieves, An Eye-Opening Exploration Into The Science And Mysteries Of Sleep,* says sleep loss makes you virtually stupid. IQ tests have shown a loss of 2 IQ points for every hour of sleep lost (assuming 8 hrs. are needed). If you get busy and lose two hours of sleep each night for 5 days, then you have lost 20 IQ points. If you are really bright, and have a 120 IQ then no big deal, you are now at the average 100 IQ. However, if you are average, you will go down to 80 which is considered retarded.

Sleep deprivation kills laboratory animals and can cause us to hallucinate and become paranoid, the good news is these effects go away with proper sleep. When we change to daylights savings time, we lose an hour of sleep and increase 7% in traffic accidents. In the Fall, we gain an hour of sleep and decrease 7% in traffic accidents.

Sleep is the time for the body's "house keeping" and repair so, if you don't get your sleep, be ready for a breakdown and major "house cleaning."

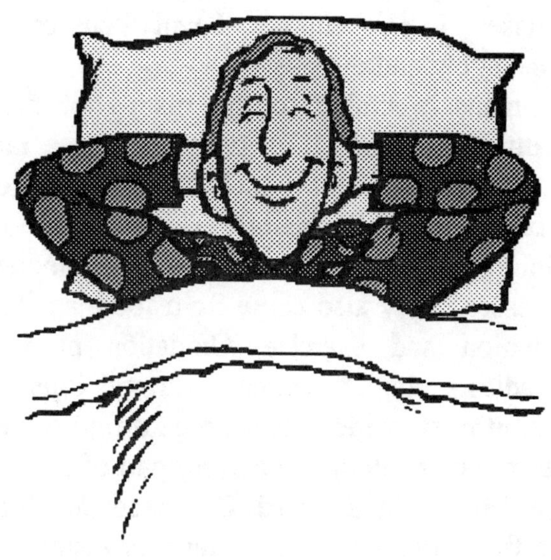

REVERSING THE AGING PROCESS

In order to reverse the aging process we need to know what causes aging. In all of my research I have found three aspects of the aging process the body, mind and spirit. In the first part of this book, I describe the rejuvenation of mind and spirit. In this section, **CREATING THE PERFECT BODY,** fitness, foods, supplements and herbs are discussed. In this chapter, I will focus on the primary cause of physical aging and disease.

Aging to humans is similar to the rusting of metals or the spoiling and rotting of food. It is caused by free radicals. Free radicals are molecules or atoms which contain unpaired electrons (Electrons normally come in pairs). These unstable molecules, usually containing oxygen are created inside our bodies in normal metabolic processes. They also come from food, smoking, alcohol, pollution, radiation and exercise. Oxidation produces several different free radicals, singlet oxygen, hydroxyl ions, hydrogen & lipid peroxides, nitrogen oxides and superoxide molecules to name a few. These free radicals can damage every part of our body.

Oxygen is a double-edged sword. It is necessary for life, yet it can initiate the free radical process, when, for instance it comes in contact with fats and oils it causes rancidity. Light strikes an oxygen molecule (a pair of oxygen atoms) and splits it apart creating a pair of singlet oxygen free radicals. Its unpaired electron then pairs with an electron stolen from a fatty acid, starting the chain reaction. Light-induced oxidation spoils oils 1000 times faster than oxidation in the dark, because light produces 1000 oxygen free radicals for every oxygen free radical produced spontaneously in the absence of light. Keep your oils and foods away from light, oxygen and heat to keep them fresh.

Note: Numbered references are at the end of the book in the reference section.

178

In an unrefined (natural) oil, natural ANTIOXIDANTS molecules such as vitamin E and others trap loose free radical electrons. Carotene and others 'quench' oxygen free radicals. Vitamin C reactivates used—up glutathione, cysteine and vitamin E, which in turn reactivates carotene and other antioxidants. Hence vitamin C plays a key role in ANTIOXIDANTS functions that prevent free radical chain reactions.

On the other hand, chlorophyll and 'pro-oxidant' metals such as iron and copper encourage free radical reactions. They help light to destroy oils even more rapidly. When oils are refined, vitamin E and carotene, as well as chlorophyll and most metals, are removed. Cheap artificial Antioxidants such as BHT, BHA and other chemical preservatives, may be added to replace the natural Antioxidants that were removed.

Does this mean we should avoid unstable oils ? Absolutely not, in fact the most disease free people have the highest level of these highly reactant oils (especially essential fatty acids EFAs) in their bodies. According to Udo Erasmus author of *Fats That Heal Fats That Kill,* "highly unsaturated fatty acids are used successfully in nutritional treatments of degenerative diseases. EFAs help bring oxygen into our system. Lack of oxygen is a key factor in degenerative diseases like cancer, aging and cardiovascular disease. Since these diseases are often associated with deficiency or functional deficiency of essential fatty acids, the supply of EFAs should not be compromised. But it must be accompanied by optimum intake of the necessary vitamins, minerals, amino acids, and antioxidants."[n]

Fire of life (the good side of oxygen)
So far it sounds like the very stuff we breathe is killing us. It is, should we now strangle ourselves? No, of course not, there is another solution. Antioxidants, also known as free radical scavengers because they neutralize free radicals.

---

[n] See the chapter: Deadly Fats vs. Healing Fats.

To understand the role of antioxidants, metabolism must be understood. Metabolism is the fire of life. Just as we may burn wood to heat our homes or petroleum products to run our cars, our bodies burn starches, oils and proteins to heat and run our bodies. The difference is, in the body things are burned more slowly and in water. The similarity is, just as the burning of wood and petroleum products produces carbon dioxide, water, pollutants and energy, so does the body. To keep the body healthy we need to burn clean fuels and keep the fire burning brightly. In a wood stove or fire place, smoky cool fires will result in clogged chimneys and possible chimney fires which may burn your house. In the body, a slow or sluggish metabolism may cause clogging of our arteries, bowels or congestion of organs and other systems° (see chapter on metabolism). Following the dietary and exercise guidelines in this book will help you burn a clean, bright, hot metabolic fire.

The down side to a hot fire is there are more sparks created. In the body the down side to a hot metabolic fire is the production of free radicals. In a fire place we use a screen to block the sparks that may pop out and burn our carpet. The screen equivalent in the body are the antioxidants, more on this later.

Excessive free radicals
In addition to the naturally produced free radicals, more may be heaped on us by the environment and poor food choices. Excessive free radicals are acquired by unnatural environmental influences such as air pollution, cigarette smoke, radiation (including sunlight), stress, pesticides, herbicides, food contaminants, processed foods, natural substances we eat including, animal products (meat and dairy), rancid foods, polyunsaturated oils and city water. These are all factors that are part of our modern life. [2]

This free radical process damages healthy cells by changing their chemical structure. Free radicals are the main cause of degenerative processes in our body (disease and aging). Free radicals can damage

---

° See the chapter: 12 Ways To Increase Your Metabolism.

cell proteins by puncturing the cell membranes and disturbing the normal nutrient/waste exchange processes. If the cells don't die from the resulting malfunction, they have lost vital hydrogen electrons, causing them to become unstable themselves. They then can create more free radicals, because they must now go and seek electrons to replenish the ones which have been taken. A potentially deadly chain reaction continues until a free radical scavenger comes along to neutralize it.

Another way to picture how free radicals affect us is to imagine a car on a highway. Suddenly, one tire rolls over a very big, sharp nail. POW! The tire blows. The car swerves out of control and crashes into another. Vehicles behind cannot stop in time, and the awful crunch of metal echoes for what seems to be forever. One tire blowout has caused a great chain reaction.

The cars represent molecules in our cells, such as proteins, enzymes, fatty acids, and genetic material. The nail is a free radical. The nail damaged the first car by popping its tire. Likewise, a free radical can damage any molecule in our body by stealing an electron. However, the car with the blowout immediately crashed into another, and a pileup resulted. So, a damaged molecule becomes a free radical, and a chain reaction begins which may involve many molecules.

Free radicals cause or greatly contribute to heart disease, cancer, arthritis and most of the diseases related to aging. Arterial disease occurs when free radicals cause a buildup of plaque along arterial walls.[3] Dr. Ishwarlal Jialal of the University of Texas Southwestern Medical Center in Dallas says that "researchers are now of the opinion that fats in the bloodstream become lodged in artery walls and begin to clog arteries only when their transporters, the lipoproteins, have chemically combined with oxygen to turn rancid."[4] Cholesterol is not so harmful until it has been oxidized.[P]

Free radicals can break vital bonds which connect atoms and molecules together, but, conversely, can also fuse other molecules

---

[P] See the Chapter: The B Vitamins.

which are not supposed to be together (cross linking). When this happens with skin tissues, stiffness and wrinkling can result. Other types of tissue breakdown attributed to free radicals can lead to cancer, inflammatory diseases, allergies and chronic illnesses.[5]

However, free radicals in minute amounts—do have their place. Natural killer (NK) cells are white blood cells which have the responsibility of destroying bacteria and virus infected cells. They use free radicals to help them accomplish this task.[2] Certain free radicals also help enzymes in the liver eliminate toxins.

ANTIOXIDANTS (free radical scavengers)—the body's natural protectors.

Antioxidants help our body combat excessive free radicals by fighting off their negative effects. Antioxidants are nutrients which donate extra hydrogen electrons to free radicals, thus neutralizing them and producing stable molecules. Antioxidant molecules give up extra electrons without turning into free radicals themselves, thus halting this harmful process. Antioxidants can be called "the body's protectors," a kind of life insurance for your cells!

The analogy of the nail on the freeway can also help illustrate how antioxidants function. If a highway sweeper had swept the nail off the road before a car could run over it, then much damage would have been avoided. Or, if the cars had tires protected with impenetrable coatings, then the nail would not be able to puncture them. So, antioxidants function as highway sweepers and tire sealant, averting potential devastation.

However, each antioxidant molecule can only neutralize one free radical. Since free radicals can multiply by the billions within only a few seconds, it is imperative that the body is constantly supplied with these vital nutrients.

Ideally, the body naturally controls the quantity of free radicals with its own antioxidant production. Problems result when the supply of free radicals exceed the body's capacity to neutralize them. Since we are all exposed to unnatural environmental influences, in one degree or another, the best precaution is to ensure a regular intake of antioxidant nutrients. Taking antioxidants is like painting your car, both processes preserve and protect.

In the body, many kinds of antioxidants protect us, including enzymes, amino acids, proteins, vitamins, minerals and other biochemicals.

Common Types Of Free Radicals	Antioxidant Protectors
Superoxides	Proanthocyanidins Quercetin, Green Tea
Peroxides	Ginkgo Biloba, Soy Schizandra, Glutathione, Cysteine, Selenium
Singlet oxygen	Lycopene
Hydroxyl	Schizandra, Melatonin

ANTIOXIDANT ENZYMES

Antioxidant enzymes are synthesized in the body. They initiate processes which ultimately channel the excessive, damaging energies of free radicals into producing harmless substances like water and ordinary oxygen. These enzymes include glutathione peroxidase, catalase, and superoxide dismutase (SOD). They are produced and function in most cells of the body. In every sense, they are a part of us. Without their protective activity, we would quickly become, quite literally, spoiled. In fact, the reason why dead flesh rots so quickly is because these enzymes no longer function.

NUTRIENTS

The most renowned antioxidants include: beta carotene (vitamin A precursor), vitamin E, vitamin C, selenium, zinc and a special group of antioxidant bioflavonoids, notably the proanthocyanidins found in the seeds and skins of blue-violet (blue berries some grapes) and red pigmented fruits. There are different types of antioxidants, however, they all work together synergistically for mutual benefit. Proanthocyanidins protect vitamin C and beta carotene, which in turn, can help extend vitamin E functions.

Antioxidant nutrients provide many benefits. They help strengthen cellular membranes, discouraging damage and permeability from pathogens such as viruses, as well as fortifying the cells against damage from active free radical molecule fragments. [6] Antioxidants help preserve the integrity of compounds such as fats, actually helping to preserve arterial walls by discouraging formation of free radicals. Vitamin E has long been revered for this purpose. They also help prevent lipid (fat) peroxidation inside the body tissues. By enhancing the vitality of cells, the aging process can be slowed.

The required antioxidant nutrient intake level for optimum nutrition will vary from one individual to another, depending upon the amount of free radical producing elements in one's life, such as exposure to pollutants, diet and even frequency of exercise.

EXERCISE

Sometimes, if you are consuming more antioxidants than your body needs, the intake can actually cause fatigue.[2] Those who participate in frequent aerobic exercise have a greater need for antioxidants, because the oxygen molecules multiply at an astonishing rate.[7] Dr. Kenneth H. Cooper, father of aerobics and author *of Antioxidant Revolution* notes that, "It has become clear that an appropriate exercise prescription becomes more complicated—especially when you take into account exposure to 'free radical triggers' such as overtraining... what is often overlooked, is that exercise must be at the center of any effective antioxidant plan. Without regular exercise, your body's internal defenses against free radicals—including natural endogenous antioxidants (those produced by the human body), such as SOD, GSH, and catalase—may become too fragile for supplements to have their effect. Studies have shown that exercising three times a week or more will induce your body to produce more of its own free radical scavengers. A weekend warrior, just working out on the weekend may be doing his body more harm than good. **Once a week workouts will produce free radicals without increasing endogenous scavengers.**

EATING

Until a few years ago the only practice that would increase the life span of experimental animals was chronic under feeding. It seems that the more you eat the faster you age. We all know some of the risks of being over weight. I believe there is more to food causing aging than just being fat.

Each time we eat, the process of digestion produces an abundance of free radicals. If we eat meat, dairy, certain fats[q] or processed foods the problem worsens. The body is designed to handle a certain amount of attack, beyond that, antioxidants are extremely important. I believe in spreading your food intake out throughout the day to decrease the chance of free radical overload. Eat six or more small meals instead of three large ones. Eat fresh raw foods first, to prepare your body with antioxidants. Imagine a freeway between the city and the suburbs. Commuters are like free radicals and the roads like antioxidants. As long as there is a steady flow, things go along smoothly. If everyone leaves at the same time, there are problems—traffic jams and pileups as mentioned earlier.

---

[q] See the chapter: Deadly Fats vs. Healing Fats.

BIOFLAVONOIDS—Amazing Antioxidants
In the 1920s, one of the greatest scientific minds of this century, Albert Szent-Gyorgi of Hungary, isolated crystals of ascorbic acid—the vitamin C we know today. At the same time, he also isolated another substance which he felt had an important nutritional function. He labeled it vitamin P (for permeability). As it turns out, the compound he found was one of a class of chemicals called bioflavonoids.

In 1993, Dutch scientists determined that people today probably consume only 23 mg of bioflavonoids each day, which is only a fifth of what we need.[30] So, we either need to eat more bioflavonoids in our food and decrease our exposure to free radicals or take supplements to protect us. I recommend 250 to 500mg/day.

Scientific interest in bioflavonoids and their effects has been booming in recent years. Scientists have now registered more than 20,000 bioflavonoids. The benefits of vitamin P are wide and varied. All are effective antioxidants. Because of the relationship between vitamin C and the bioflavonoids, include the whole fruit such as acerola cherries and the white tissue beneath the skin of citrus fruit. These should be present for optimal benefits. A few specific bioflavonoids have important biological functions, as noted below.

Quercetin—The Antioxidant King
Quercetin has been one of the most widely studied bioflavonoids in recent years. This bioflavonoid is one of the most common compounds in nature and is present in a wide variety of the natural foods such as onions, fruits and vegetables.

Quercetin is an amazing compound. In therapeutic settings, scientists have seen that it has a great, positive effect on a variety of disorders. Quercetin researchers have seen positive effects from quercetin in: Breast cancer therapy;[8] Stomach cancer treatment;[9] General cancer research;[10] Lessen the side effects from radiation therapy;[11] Help treat inflammation of the parotid glands;[12] As an active ingredient in two traditional remedies to treat diarrhea;[13,14] Assisting the effectiveness of anti-viral treatments;[15] May help to lessen diabetic complications;[16] May help to lessen certain heart arrhythmias.[17]

Scientists have one concern about quercetin—what effect large doses of this bioflavonoid would do to a person over the long term. Some concern has been raised that it interacts with DNA.[18] To be safe, the amount of quercetin consumed in formulations should be in the same range as what you would receive if you consumed a proper diet based on fruits and vegetables.

There is much to be optimistic about. You might even call quercetin the "king of the antioxidants" because the results of the tests have been so positive. It could become the vitamin C of the next century.

Hesperidin—A study of 100 people in Italy showed that a flavonoid mix containing hesperidin "increases to a large extent the capillary resistance in patients with abnormal capillary fragility without significant side effects."[19] A study showed that hesperidin from oranges "possesses significant anti-inflammatory and analgesic effects."[20]

Naringin—A study shows that high doses of naringin seems to help protect against ulcers caused by alcohol consumption.[21] One study says that grapefruit juice contains a great deal of naringin and other related compounds. This fact "may be of relevance to cancer chemoprevention."[22]

Rutin—Oriental scientists tested seven flavonoids as scavengers of super oxides, and rutin was the most effective. Naringin and quercetin tied for second.[23] Rutin, like naringin, was shown to have a positive effect in preventing damage to the stomach from alcohol consumption.[24] Along with quercetin and silymarin, rutin was seen to be a possible "chemopreventative agent" in the study of cancer of the trachea.[25]

Milk Thistle (Silymarin the essential component of milk thistle)—Milk thistle is the greatest liver protector and regenerator. Liver disease is one of America's greatest health problems, affecting 25 million people. It is the leading cause of death for people between the ages of 25 and 59. The liver is the largest internal organ in our bodies. It's primary purpose is to remove or detoxify poisons, drugs, alcohol and other harmful chemicals. It also regulates much of our metabolism. In this technological era we are bombarded with toxic pollution and both prescription and over the counter drugs. Without the liver these would kill us. An over dose of acetaminophen can irreversibly damage the liver and cause a slow painful death similar to the death cased by the Amanita "death cap" mushroom. The Amanita is so liver toxic that only 30–40% of its victims survive with standard treatment.

Dr. G. Vogel treated 60 patients suffering with severe Amanita poisoning with milk thistle extract and every single person survived. Numerous studies have shown that milk thistle with 80% silymarin, to be helpful in treating several types of hepatitis and liver disease.

I take milk thistle two to three times a day to protect the most important detoxifying organ in my body.

Bilberry Extract—Bilberry is the antioxidant for the eyes, circulation and connective tissue. In over 70 clinical trials, involving people from all walks of life, bilberry has been shown to improve eyesight and relieve eyestrain. According to *The Textbook of Natural Medicine*, bilberry anthocyanosides are important in prevention and/or treatment of glaucoma, cataracts, macular degeneration, diabetic retinopathy, nightblindness and retinitis pigmentosa. Quite simply, bilberry is the free radical scavenger for the eyes.

Bilberry has also been shown to be helpful in small and large vessel diseases including arteriosclerosis, varicose veins and microvascular disease (capillary function).

Hawthorn Extract—Hawthorn (crataegus oxyacantha) is one of the most popular heart remedies in Europe where its efficacy is well-researched and proven.

For example, a 1981 German study, involving over 6,000 patients, found that hawthorn significantly improves the heart's function and health. In other studies hawthorn reduced high blood pressure, angina attacks, and serum cholesterol.

According to Rudolf Weiss, M.D., hawthorn works by increasing coronary blood flow, improving cardiac function and by reducing or helping to prevent cardiac arrhythmias. Dr. Weiss goes on to explain that hawthorn is "completely safe for long-term use." In fact, the herb works best when it's used for several weeks to several months.

Hawthorn's health benefits are attributed to natural, healing substances (biologically active flavonoids) extracted from leaves and berries. The highest quality hawthorn supplement available is a concentrated extract guaranteed to contain 1.8% vitexin–2'–rhamnoside. The typical dosage is 100–200 mg daily.

Hawthorn is especially helpful when taken with other healing herbs such as ginkgo biloba. According to Dr. Weiss, hawthorn's action is directed mainly toward the coronary vessels, while ginkgo biloba, bilberry and garlic act mainly on peripheral vessels.

Proanthocyanidins

The most famous bioflavonoid members in today's news are the leucoanthocyanins, also known as proanthocyanidins or pycnogenols. The word terms in proanthocyanidin have the following meanings: PRO: The prefix pro means before. When you have a pro-vitamin, you can break it apart to make a vitamin. Pro-vitamin C breaks into vitamin C and an indole. ANTHO: This root word means flower. Someone with anthophobia is afraid of flowers. CYAN: This root word means color. As any printer knows, cyan (along with yellow, magenta, and black) is one of the four colors used in printing magazines. In this case, cyan seems to mean more simply, color. IDINS: This root word makes it a part of a family. Just as a person from Japan is Japanese, so are nutrients from the anthocyan family—anthocyanidins. Therefore, proanthocyanidins are wonderful nutrients that create the color of flowers and other plants. These beautiful chemicals are also good for you. They are some of the best antioxidants available.

Proanthocyanidins were first extracted from pine tree bark by Dr. Jacques Masquelier, a French researcher. Dr. Masquelier coined the term "pycnogenols" to describe the proanthocyanidins extracted from the bark. His interest in these bioflavonoids led him to subsequently seek a richer and more widely available source of proanthocyanidins. When he researched the Vitas Vinifera species of grape, he knew that he had discovered what he was looking for. Since then, the majority of the clinical and experimental studies have been conducted using grape seed extract, and the results extrapolated to the earlier pine bark extract.

Dr. Masquelier endorses the grape seed extract over the pine bark extract as a more effective and a better source of the proanthocyanidins.[27] Grape seed contains 92 to 95 percent proanthocyanidins, compared to 80 to 85 percent in pine bark.

Studies report the antioxidative potency of proanthocyanidins as being remarkably 20 to 50 times more potent than vitamin E. Other studies indicate that proanthocyanidins seem to help nutritionally support connective tissues and capillaries.[28, 29]

Arthritis & Glucosamine

According to some estimates, osteoarthritis affects more than half of the adult population.[1] In this condition the affected joints undergo degenerative changes, including loss of articular cartilage. Osteoarthritis is the most common form of arthritis, and its exact cause is unknown. The most common treatments for this disorder are analgesics and anti-inflammatory agents. However, they do nothing to correct the underlying degenerative process and only provide relief from pain. In fact, there is evidence that they tend to further impair cartilage metabolism, possibly making the long-term situation worse.[2]

Glucosamine is an amino-monosaccharide naturally present in the body and cartilage, where it is a component of different types of glycosaminoglycans of the matrix of cartilage.[3] Its main physiological role is to stimulate proteoglycan synthesis, for which it represents one of the essential substrates. Studies have suggested that altered glucosamine metabolism plays a role in the development of osteoarthritis,[4] and numerous clinical studies have been published examining the effect of glucosamine supplementation on osteoarthritis.

In the early 1980's, a series of published studies documented the effects of glucosamine sulfate on human patients with osteoarthritis. To begin with, glucosamine treatment was compared with an Italian anti-arthritic drug which was claimed to be particularly useful for arthritis flare-ups.[5] During the initial week of treatment no significant difference in effectiveness between the compounds was demonstrated, and each symptom improved significantly. The following two weeks, however, showed a significant difference between the treatments. Whereas the glucosamine group continued to improve, the comparison groups symptom scores rose to almost pretreatment levels. The results led the researchers to conclude that treatment with glucosamine, "effectively managed the symptoms of osteoarthritis and succeeded in improving articular function, as suggested by the basic biochemical and pharmacological investigations." That same year a longer, double-blind study in established osteoarthritis demonstrated that over a 6 to 8 week period glucosamine sulfate were significantly more effective than a placebo.[6] The results included improvements in articular pain, joint tenderness, and restricted movement. Additionally, patients given glucosamine experienced an earlier alleviation of symptoms compared to the placebo group. Importantly, no adverse reactions or variations in laboratory tests was recorded. These impressive results culminated with the author's conclusion that, "glucosamine sulfate is a drug of first choice for the basic treatment of patients with osteoarthritis."

Two years later, a double-blind clinical evaluation of glucosamine sulfate was carried out by comparing it with ibuprofen, a commonly prescribed and recommended treatment for osteoarthritis.[7] Although ibuprofen and glucosamine were both well tolerated, several interesting differences were observed. While ibuprofen resulted in faster pain relief during the first two weeks of the study, glucosamine was significantly more effective by the eighth week. Additionally, the attending physicians, who where unaware of which patients received which compound, showed a significant preference for glucosamine over ibuprofen. The authors concluded that the best therapeutic results may be obtained by combining an anti-inflammatory (like ibuprofen) with glucosamine for the initial two weeks of treatment, followed by maintenance therapy with glucosamine alone.

During the early 1990's, a series of papers were published on research conducted by the Italian pharmaceutical company that markets glucosamine sulfate preparations in Italy and other countries around the world.[8] These papers demonstrated the effectiveness of glucosamine sulfate in numerous animal models of arthritis and inflammation. The conclusion of these studies was that glucosamine has significant activity in many different animal models of arthritis and inflammation. Most importantly, glucosamine showed much lower toxicity than traditional anti-arthritic drugs, leading the authors to comment that because "the large therapeutic margin in experimental subacute and chronic inflammatory and arthritic models, and the safety in prolonged oral administration, it is justified to classify glucosamine sulfate as a potential disease-modifying drug for long-term treatments of osteoarthritis and other rheumatic disorders."

In 1991, an interesting study on the effect of N-acetylglucosamine on cartilage degeneration in rats was published.[9] It showed that N-acetylglucosamine given orally not only had a positive effect on the production of cartilage, but also increased the incorporation of glucosamine into the cartilage. N-acetylglucosamine also appeared to inhibit subsequent degenerative changes in non-arthritic joints, a common progression in arthritis.

Using Glucosamine

While most clinical trials have utilized glucosamine sulfate, the fact that some people may lack the ability to efficiently convert glucosamine into N-acetylglucosamine (a necessary step in the production of cartilage) suggests that a combination of glucosamine sulfate and N-acetylglucosamine may be more effective. Most studies have utilized daily dosages of 500 milligrams given in three divided doses. However, glucosamine sulfate has also been shown to be effective when given intermittently as a twice a week treatment.[10] Thus, some experimentation may be necessary to find the best treatment regimen. Additionally, since anti-inflammatory agents seem to complement glucosamine supplements by providing short-term relief from pain, the use of agents such as copper salicylate along with glucosamine sulfate and N-acetylglucosamine may provide additional benefits.

Tea the ancient longevity drink—Several studies of thousands of people have shown tea to be life extending and disease preventing. Dr. John Weisburger a prominent cancer researcher drinks about five cups a day. He claims it is as powerful as two fruits or vegetables in its antioxidant power. Tea is chalked full of antioxidant polyphenols, such as quercetin and catechins. Italian researchers have shown that tea peps up the antioxidant activity of the blood close to 50% for eighty minutes. The antioxidant activity began at thirty minutes after consuming a cup of green tea and fifty minutes after consuming black tea.

Both green and black tea kill the bacteria that causes gum disease and cavities. This is good not only for kids but also for adults. According to Alan Winter, DDS –almost all tooth loss after the age of forty is caused by gum disease–and nearly 80% of people over forty have some gum disease.

Beer, Wine and Cocoa—contain phenols that help prevent the oxidation of LDL cholesterol.[r] Phenols are high in red wine and dark beers. Alcohol by itself is also beneficial in "thinning" the blood. More than two drinks per day increases the risk for other diseases. Women have increased risk of breast cancer with one or more alcoholic drinks per day. **I do not recommend starting to drink beer or wine if you don't already drink alcoholic beverages.** However, if you do drink, stick with red wine and dark beer and drink moderately.

Attention chocoholics! Cocoa seems to have the same health benefits as wine and beer without the alcohol. Researchers from my alma mater, the University of California at Davis have reported the benefits of red wine in 1993 and in September of 1996 are reporting similar benefits for chocolate. When placed in a test tube, cocoa phenols inhibited LDL oxidation by 75 percent, while a similar concentration of red wine phenols reduced harmful oxidation by 37 to 65 percent.

Another health benefit of cocoa, is that like tea it helps prevent cavities. Your best source of healthy cocoa is pure low-fat cocoa powder.[s] If you are going to eat chocolate bars, check the ingredients. Beware of unhealthy fats[t] and sugars. Cocoa butter is

---

[r] It is the oxidized LDL cholesterol that causes most cardiovascular diseases.

[s] Wonderslim® makes this for questions and recipes call 1-800 497-6595.

[t] See the chapter: Deadly Fats vs. Healing Fats.

neutral, it doesn't affect cholesterol levels, it will however, make you fat if you eat too much.[u]

Vegetable/Fruit pills—are generally dried up powdered vegetables or fruit. Example, one pill claimed these ingredients: Tomato Concentrate (1% Lycopenes) 20mg. which means it actually has 0.2 mg of lycopenes. You would have to eat over 10,000 pills to get the amount contained in one small tomato; Soy Extract (1% Isoflavones) 20 mg or 0.2mg. of Isoflavones. 200 pills would equal the Isoflavone content of a 4 oz slice of tofu or a cup of soy milk.

OTHER SUPER FOODS
Soy products—Tofu has its own chapter.
Flaxseed—has its own chapter.
Garlic—has its own chapter.
Tomato—one tomato (100 grams) has 3 grams (3,000 mgs) of lycopene plus 10,000 other phytonutrients.
Broccoli—an amazing powerhouse of nutrition, loaded with antioxidants: sulforaphane,[v] vitamin C, beta carotene, quercetin, indoles, glutathione, chromium and other important minerals.
Citrus fruit—the orange has every class of anticancer inhibitor known, including carotenoids, terpenes (liminene), flavonoids and vitamin C. Grapefruit has its own anti-aging nutrients including glutathione and a unique fiber that helps reverse atherosclerosis. Remember that the whole raw fruit is better than juice. Bottled juice has minimal benefits if any because it has been cooked and is diluted with about 90% sugar water (corn syrup).

Glutathione—The body's master antioxidant. Blood glutathione levels are used as a biochemical index of aging, in other words, your

---

[u] Two other healthy sources of cocoa are: Sunspire® chocolate chips and Pamelas™ Ultra Chocolate Brownie mix.
[v] Sulforaphane causes carcinogens to be rejected by cells. Also high in other cruciferous vegetables eg. cabbage, cauliflower, Brussel sprouts and turnips.

blood level of glutathione shows your biological age. Supplements and high glutathione foods such as avocados and watermelon only work on the food in the G.I. tract, it is not well absorbed. The best way to increase it is to take the amino acid L-cysteine 500mg with 2 grams of vitamin C, 100 mcg of selenium (2-3 Brazil nuts) and the amino acid glutamine (take 3 gms or up to 20 gms when ill or stressed).

Coenzyme Q10—also known as ubiquinone, is a micronutrient essential to all human life. This naturally occurring nutrient is a cofactor in the electron transport system from which all of the body's energy is derived. CoQ10 is, therefore, absolutely essential for helping the body produce energy at the cellular level where it regulates the intake of oxygen. CoQ10 supplies the very "spark of life" that creates the required energy for all human cells. Without sufficient CoQ10 we simply would not have enough energy to survive.

Most people become deficient in CoQ10 during times of illness, environmental stress or aging. For example, by the time we reach 60 years of age nearly 75% of our CoQ10 levels are depleted. Dietary supplementation, nevertheless, helps restore youthful levels of this vital nutrient. Half of the people who are obese are deficient in CoQ10. When the deficient group was given only 30 mgs. per day they lost more than twice the weight as the non deficient group.

CoQ10 is a popular supplement in Japan, it is taken by over 15 million people every day. What's more, scientific research with this popular nutrient has been so impressive that CoQ10 is often referred to as a "miracle nutrient" in the world of conservative science. As further testimony to the importance of this remarkable substance scientists have received top honors for their work with CoQ10 including Peter Mitchell (Nobel Prize winner) and Dr. Karl Folkers (winner of the coveted Priestly Medal of Honor). Julian Whitaker, M.D., author and founder of the Whitaker Wellness Institute wrote a letter to Dr. Peter Gott, M.D. (syndicated newspaper columnist). Dr. Gott had denounced the use of CoQ10. Dr. Whitaker said:

Dear Dr. Gott,

At first I was incredulous, then alarmed by your comments on coenzyme Q10.

I have been practicing medicine in California for twenty years and have been dispensing, prescribing, and recommending coenzyme Q10 daily for over a decade. A health food store close to me has seven brands of high-quality coenzyme Q10, which are made in Japan.

Coenzyme Q10 is not a "nontraditional" treatment of cardiomyopathy; it is the most powerful treatment of cardiomyopathy available. It increases the survival rate of cardiomyopathy patients tenfold compared to the combined therapy of ACE inhibitors, diuretics, and Lanoxin. No university centers are looking at coenzyme Q10, primarily because of the imposing procedures of the Food and Drug Administration. Per Langsjoen, M.D., a cardiologist in Tyler, Texas, has been prescribing and publishing information on coenzyme Q10 for years. He knows of no other efforts in this country.

We are rapidly marching towards an allopathic dark age in which information not even remotely related to fact is "generated" to serve allopathic medical dogma. Doctors will become even more like robots, exhibiting no signs of independent thought. Your piece on coenzyme Q10 is testimony that perhaps you have already arrived.

For your reader with cardiomyopathy who inquired about coenzyme Q10, you need to set the record straight and inform her that she can get it at a health food store, if she so desires. To withhold this information from her is unreasonable, unethical, and will facilitate her demise, and potentially that of many others. However, since coenzyme Q10 is a nutrient, not a drug, it is not "politically correct" to mention anything positive about it, and the mention of health food stores is strictly forbidden.

What are you going to do?

According to the best-selling book, *The Miracle Nutrient CoQ10*, by Emile G. Bliznakov, M.D., and medical writer Gerald L. Hunt, extensive research with CoQ10 has revealed the following potential benefits:
• Helps boost energy levels and endurance;
• Enhances the immune system;
• Strengthens and protects the heart;
• Helps normalize blood pressure;
• Reverses periodontal (gum) disease;
• Aids in weight loss without dieting;
• Improves response to chemotherapy;
• Protects against free-radical toxins;
• Helps reverse the effects of aging naturally.

Every cell in your body contains a tiny power plant (mitochondrion), that needs fuel to produce energy for everything you do. This fuel is oxygen.

That's why CoQ10 is so important. It regulates the flow of oxygen moving in and out of the cell's power plant. In this way CoQ10 acts like a spark plug in a car providing the necessary spark for the engine's ignition. So, just like a car that can't function without a spark plug, the body's cellular power plants can't function without CoQ10.

A **dec**line or disruption in the body's CoQ10 levels can lead to illness. For example, Dr. Karl Folkers says that when CoQ10 levels drop below 75% (a 25% deficiency) we may become ill. He goes on to say that when CoQ10 levels drop below 25% (a 75% deficiency) death occurs.

HORMONES

Melatonin—may be the most powerful hydroxyl radical antioxidant discovered to date.

In reality, it makes perfect sense, since melatonin is produced at night during the body's restore and repair cycle. In fact, melatonin appears to be particularly important in the protection of DNA against free radical attack. And so, this bit player of human physiology is now seen as one of your body's most important anti-cancer defenses.

It's even more than that. The protection of DNA, the cell's blueprint, is the protection of life. That's why every living thing produces melatonin. We also know that melatonin production decreases as we age, and this decline may be a major factor in the increased risk for cancer.

DHEA: THE MOTHER HORMONE

This information is from ABC's Good Morning America:

"Dubbed the "mother of all hormones" (its "offspring" include the sex hormones estrogen and androgens), DHEA may also buffer the effects of stress hormones and prevent age-related diseases. "When you put the pieces together," says Stanford University biologist Robert Sapolsky, Ph.D., "DHEA levels are a fairly significant predictor of longevity."

Low DHEA has been linked to a murderer's row of diseases, including breast cancer, obesity, high cholesterol, hypertension and heart disease. Even under normal circumstances, DHEA levels decline by as much as 75 percent between early adulthood and old age.

In animals, DHEA replacement works wonders, fighting obesity, protecting against diabetes, sharpening memory and warding off infectious diseases. In humans, DHEA supplementation is controversial. Though it's long been used in Europe as an anti-obesity and anti-aging drug, some scientists warn high doses may lead to liver damage and excessive testosterone levels.

On the plus side, when Samuel S.C. Yen, M.D., and his colleagues at the University of California School of Medicine in La Jolla gave 50 mg of DHEA daily for six months to 13 men and 17 women ages 40 to 70. They reported "a remarkable increase" in physical and psychological well-being, deeper sleep and an improved ability to handle stress. If you're interested, talk to your doctor. DHEA is powerful stuff—ill advised for do-it-yourselfers.

From Holistic Health News written by Ray Gebauer:

What single weakness would you guess that aging, cancer, heart disease, diabetes, obesity, osteoporosis and chronic fatigue have in common? According to Dr. Julian Whitaker's Health and Healing Newsletter (Feb./1994), it appears that having low blood levels of DHEA is the common factor!

DHEA (dehydroepiandrosterone), produced by your adrenal glands, is the most dominant hormone in your body. Dr. William Regelson, the most noted of DHEA researchers, calls it the "mother hormone" because your body converts it upon demand into hormones it needs, such as estrogen, testosterone and adrenaline.

Blood levels of DHEA peak around age 20. It is the only hormone that declines in a linear fashion in both sexes continuously after age 20-25, making it one of the most reliable markers of aging. Levels fall to 0-5% in the last year of life! Its decline signals age-related diseases. According to Dr. Deepak Chopra, in his best selling book, *Ageless Body, Timeless Mind*, the more stress you have, the lower your blood levels of DHEA are, since stress depletes your reservoir of DHEA.

There have been over 40,000 medical studies and articles on DHEA. In one study on 5,000 apparently healthy women, it was discovered that 100% of the women that developed and died of breast cancer had blood levels of DHEA less than 10% of the norm for their age group. These women had subnormal DHEA levels up to nine years before their cancer was diagnosed. Yet 100% of the women with higher-than-average levels of DHEA remained cancer free. In a subsequent study, DHEA was given to rats genetically bred to always develop breast cancer. Amazingly, DHEA blocked it 100% of the time. None of the rats given DHEA got cancer!

Elizabeth Barrett-Connor, M.D., from the Department of Community and Family Medicine at the University of California School of Medicine in San Diego, tracked DHEA levels in 242 men ages 50 to 79 for twelve years. She found that 48% reduction in cardiovascular disease and a 36% reduction of mortality from any cause was correlated to a 100 microgram-per-deciliter increase in DHEA sulfate blood levels. In the New England Journal of Medicine, she and other researchers concluded that even in people without heart disease, DHEA seems to protect against early death.

A 1988 study was done at John Hopkins Medical Institute in which rabbits with severe arteriosclerosis were treated with DHEA. They had an almost 50% reduction in plaque size.

Arthur Schwartz, a researcher at Temple University in Philadelphia, found that DHEA blocks an enzyme called G-6PD that promotes cancer-cell division, as well as fat production. "There isn't any question," Schwartz says, "DHEA is a very effective anti-obesity agent." In mice, it gives almost a 50% reduction in excess fat, according to Norman Applezweig of Progenics, Inc.

In fact, DHEA appears to be the first substance that when laboratory tested, caused the loss of fat (as opposed to mere weight loss due to the breakdown of primary lean muscle tissue or fluid loss) without changing eating habits. Calories consumed were simply converted to heat rather than stored as fat. At the same time, it helps the body to produce lean muscle tissue.

In the January 1994 issue of Health Revelation, Dr. Robert Atkins states that DHEA has been shown to improve memory in aging mice. There has been very active ongoing research on using

DHEA against Alzheimer's disease. One study showed blood levels of DHEA in a group of Alzheimer's patients to be 48% lower than the control group.

Dr. Kenneth Bonnet, a research scientist in the Department of Psychiatry at New York University School of Medicine, describes detailed testing with a 47-year-old woman with lifelong multiple learning disabilities and low memory retention. Within one week of low doses of DHEA, the patient showed an improvement in recall ability and was sleeping better. The woman also reported feeling an increase in clear thinking and her ability to remember. After one month, a higher dose of DHEA was given to the woman. Testing showed a more advanced ability to recall with an increase in long-term memory. Also, for the first time in her 47 years of life, she was able to begin and continue to run a small business!

I am happy to report that as of September 1996 DHEA is available over the counter. I personally take 50mg. every morning.

Synthetic Foods And Drugs
Synthetic substances like Nutrasweet, Olestra, prescription and non-prescription drugs, can mimic some effects of natural substances in our body but are in other ways quite different from natural substances. They are likely to 'misfit' our body's enzyme structure and effectively throw a monkey wrench into our body's metabolism. They might produce more free radicals or block the absorption of antioxidants. Olestra blocks the absorption of fat soluble vitamins such as vitamins A, E, D and K. Other synthetic substances use up more of our body's antioxidant nutrient defenses and lead to degenerative diseases. The 'side effects' of many prescription drugs and the toxic effects of many pesticides and poisons are caused by the free radical chain reactions they initiate.

Bottom line:

1. Stick to a mostly vegetarian diet.

2. Eat more than 50% of your foods raw.

3. Exercise more than three times per week, include resistance training.

4. Supplement your diet with vitamins, minerals, herbs and antioxidants.

5. Develop a healthy emotional and spiritual outlook. A counselor can often be of great assistance.

6. Avoid toxins.

7. Under eat.

8. Drink tea throughout the day.

9. Have a customized health program designed for you by someone who knows and understands the principles of this book.

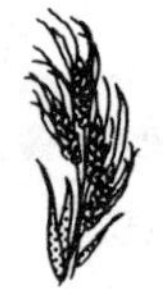

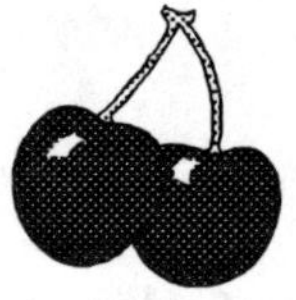

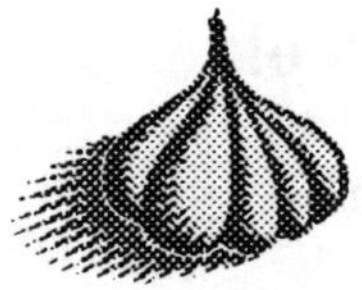

FOODS, SUPPLEMENTS AND SPICES

Milk, Calcium, and Bone Density, A Catch-22
by Charles R. Attwood, M.D., F.A.A.P.
used with permission

A note from the school dietitian was handed to me by a young mother of a 7 year old boy. "Billy's diet has come to our attention," it read, "because he no longer selects milk in the cafeteria." He had recently given up milk at my suggestion because it worsened his asthma and eczema. The note went on to conclude, "Milk is absolutely necessary for protein and calcium!" This last sentence was heavily underlined. I quickly realized how concerned Billy's mother was, because there was also a history of osteoporosis among several elderly members of her family.

This dilemma is encountered most frequently by families who are trying to reduce saturated fat and animal proteins in their diets. They've read that both may increase the risk of heart disease and certain cancers, but worry about calcium balance and bone density if milk, the chief source of saturated fat for children, is discontinued. I often reassure concerned parents that some bowing of their child's legs is normal up to the age of 3, and is not due to a calcium deficiency or rickets. Dental decay in early childhood, causes the same concern, but ironically it is partially due to the frequent bathing of the teeth with milk, rather than a calcium deficiency.

Why is this paranoia so common among Americans? **The milk-calcium-bone density myth has been created and perpetuated by the intense lobbying of the dairy industry** throughout the lifetimes of most adults living today. Throughout kindergarten and grade school, most of the nutrition teaching aids were supplied by the American Dairy Council. As a result, most parents, teachers, doctors, lawyers, judges, and significantly, members of congress grew up with the not unbiased view that milk is a necessary and wholesome food for both children and adults.

The council's most effective campaign tool has been to link milk, calcium, and bone density.

To further confuse the consumer, milk and infant formulas have been fortified with vitamin D, which is necessary for proper calcium absorption. It may also be obtained by eating sardines, herring, salmon, tuna, egg yolk, and fish oils. However, none of these are necessary, because it's manufactured in adequate amounts by exposure to as little as 10-15 minutes of sunlight about three times a week. Rickets may be prevented in children getting no sunlight—such as the totally disabled, by a vitamin D supplement, if the parents do not wish to fed them fortified milk.

The true connection between milk and strong bones isn't exactly what the dairy industry has been telling us all these years. Calcium balance, the relationship between the intake and loss of the mineral determines bone density, mostly during childhood and adolescence. Good bone density attained by the age of 18 usually lasts a lifetime for people consuming a balanced plant-based diet and remaining physically active. **Milk and other dairy products, although rich in calcium, are high in animal protein, which has been shown to create calcium loss through the urinary tract.** A 1994 National Institutes of Health Consensus Conference concluded that calcium balance and bone density depended at least 30 percent on the ratio of intake to loss, not on calcium intake alone. According to a report in *Science* magazine in 1986, evidence is accumulating that calcium intake (considered alone) is not related to bone density This may explain why countries consuming the most milk also have the highest incidence of osteoporosis. Exceptions exist, but a common determining factor seems to be the high protein consumption in populations who require very high levels of calcium intake. For instance, the RDA of calcium in the United States is up to 1,200 mg. daily. This is much higher than the World Health Organization's recommendation of 500 mg. for children and 800 mg for adults. Areas of the world where dietary protein is very low have low national recommendations. In

Thailand, for example, the recommended daily intake of calcium is only 400 mg. for all ages. Elderly South African Bantu women, who consume a very low protein diet (50 grams daily, compared with 91 grams for Americans) and only 450 mg. calcium daily, have no osteoporosis despite the calcium drain of nursing an average of 10 children. On the other hand, Eskimos, consuming a very high protein diet (250-400 grams) of fish, and a calcium intake of over 2,000 mg daily, have the highest rate of osteoporosis in the world!

Now, let's take a new look at milk and dairy products as a calcium source, regardless of their protein content. Calcium expressed as mg. per 100 calories instead of per gram show milk and cheese at the bottom of the list and green vegetables at the top (see chart).

Calcium in Milligrams per 100 Calories	
Arugula	1,300
Watercress	800
Turnip greens	650
Collard green	548
Mustard green	490
Spinach	450
Broccoli	387
Swiss cheese	250
Milk (2-percent)	245
Green onions	240
Okra	213
Cabbage	196
Whole milk	190
Cheddar cheese	179
American cheese	160

At first glance, one may conclude, "but I would have to eat so much more spinach or kale to get adequate calcium." Not so, individuals on a plant-based diet generally eat as many total calories as meat and dairy-eaters. In other words, adequate amounts of **vegetables are better sources of calcium than milk and cheese**.[w] Also, consider that a cup of broccoli contains about the same amount of calcium as a cup of milk. But wait! Haven't we been told that many green vegetables contain oxalic acid, which reduces the absorption of their calcium. This too, has been exaggerated by the dairy lobby. A 1990 report in the American Journal of Clinical Nutrition concluded that greens such as broccoli and kale have high levels of calcium which is absorbed at least as well of that in milk. Excellent calcium balance on a non-dairy diet is easily attained because ALL vegetables and legumes contain calcium, and collectively it's more than adequate. This calcium stays in the bones, unlike much of that from the high protein-containing dairy products.

Now it begins to make sense. In cultures where the most protein is consumed, the calcium requirement for good bone density and protection against osteoporosis may be **unattainably** high, without supplements—it's a Catch-22. But for the majority of the world population, and among those consuming a plant-based diet in Western countries, calcium requirements for normal bone density are easily obtained without milk or other dairy products. Milk, it now seems clear, is not the solution to the malady of poor bone density. It may be a part of the problem.

Charles R. Attwood, M.D., F.A.A.P., a pediatrician based in Crowley, Louisiana, is the author of Dr. Attwood's Low-Fat Prescription For Kids (Viking). It represents one diet for the whole family. He is a regular columnist for New Century Nutrition. His new audio series, The Gold Standard Diet, is produced by Knowledge Products (1-888-TOP-DIET)

I agree whole heartedly with Dr. Attwood's condemnation of milk, **It does not do a body good!**

---

[w] Where do you think the cows got their calcium?

It is interesting to note that humans are the only animal species that continues to drink milk past infancy and humans are the only animals that drink another species milk. Cow's milk is quite different in composition compared to human milk—cow's milk is designed to take a baby calf and create a several ton animal in months. Drink milk and look like a cow.

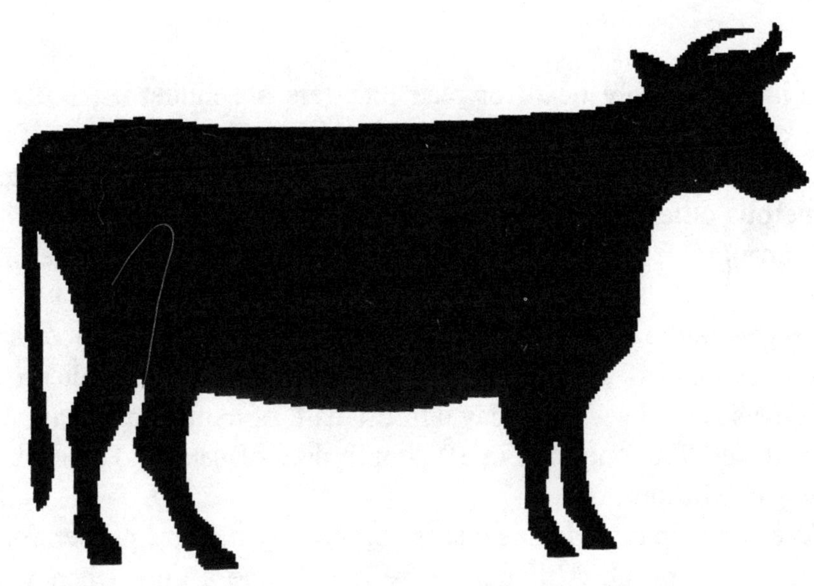

DEADLY FATS VS. HEALING FATS

You have probably heard or read that fats are killing us, but did you know that it is only certain kinds of fat. The facts are in; fats can also heal us. The high incidence of heart disease, cancer and numerous other diseases is not caused only by the amount of fat we consume. It is the *type of fat* we eat and a deficiency of healing fats.

Degenerative diseases that involve fat have rapidly increased since 1900. In 1900, only one in seven people died of cardiovascular disease. Today almost half of Americans will die from it. In 1900, only one in 30 people died of cancer. Today it is nearly one in four.

We can help reverse this disease process by making proper food choices, to a point. Although, there does come a time when vital organs are so severely damaged they cannot recover. In other words, reversal of degeneration is no longer possible. Now is the time to make some changes in your eating habits. You may decide to avoid the deadly fats or add the healing ones to your diet. The choice is yours and the knowledge to choose is what I will emphasize in this chapter.

Even genetic diseases that affect 1 in 200 of us, may not be curable but our health can still be improved with proper nutrition.

Depression and mental health can be greatly improved with proper eating.

Low Fat Diets Will Not Save Us

You may already be aware that the U.S. Department of Health and Agriculture has recommended that all Americans over the age of two should decrease their fat intake to below 30% of their daily calories, and their saturated fat intake to below 10%. Unfortunately, following this recommendation will not save you from degenerative diseases. Research reveals that a low fat diet may actually speed the degenerative process. This is because many low fat diets are low in health promoting fats as well as being high in damaging ones.

In order to understand the difference between good and bad fats we need to know the definition of fat. Fats and oils are lipids. They are made of carbon, hydrogen and oxygen. Both plants and animals produce fats. Fats may be saturated or unsaturated. Unsaturated fats may be monounsaturated (i.e. olive oil - and have one double bond or kink in their molecular structure), polyunsaturated (i.e. corn or safflower oil - usually having two double bonds or kinks), and superunsaturated (i.e. flax seed and fish oils - having three or more double bonds or kinks).

If the fat or oil is solid at room temperature it is deadly.

Saturated fats are most commonly found in animal products. Whether a fat is health promoting or disease producing is determined by how they stack up. Also, properties of fats (how they function in our bodies) is determined in part by their molecular structure. This structure can be described as caterpillar shape. Unsaturated fats have kinks and bends everywhere there is a double bond (an unsaturated spot). This keeps them from stacking neatly together and is why they are liquid at room temperature. Saturated fats are straight so they stack neatly together, are

213

relatively non-reactive and are solid at room temperature. For example, lard and butter are saturated animal fats; coconut and palm oil are saturated vegetable fats. Saturated fats are also much more stable than the unsaturated fats and go rancid less easily. This is why the food industry prefers to use saturated fats. The shelf life of foods with saturated fats is much longer.

Deadly Trans-Fats

Have you noticed that the food industry has decreased its use of animal fats to make their products seem more healthy? Don't let that fool you. They have simply replaced them with something even more deadly—partially hydrogenated vegetable oils. These oils are made by forcing hydrogen atoms into the fats' molecular structure and thus disrupting the double bonds that shape the molecule. Dozens of unnatural fats are made by hydrogenation and many of them are toxic to the body. Perhaps, the worst of these is the trans-fats. Trans-fats are formed at high temperatures creating a twist around the double bond, rendering a straighter, less biologically active substance. This 180° twist drastically changes its chemical properties, its biological activity and how it functions in the body. Fats from plant sources are in a "cis" molecular structure. This structure creates a bend and makes this oil more biologically active.

The trans-fats disrupt the body's metabolism, in part, by changing the permeability of all the cells in our body. Like saturated fat, trans-fats are solid at body temperature. When our cell membranes pick up too many of these, they harden like lard and the cell's permeability changes. Permeability determines what substances come into or out of our cells. Toxic substances may be let in, or not allowed to be removed from our cells. Scientists have known this for 20 years, yet haven't been concerned because the "Standard American Diet" (SAD) contains only 3-4% of calories as trans-fats. While this amount was felt to be negligible, animal studies have shown gross cell abnormalities with just a little over

214

4%. Human studies have shown elevations in the "bad" LDL cholesterol in only three weeks of eating a diet high in trans-fats. The amount of trans-fats in most Americans' diets is rising rapidly.

Another factor to consider is that a cell with fluid membranes will be much more likely to bring in and metabolize excess sugars, fats and toxins. This helps to keep our blood clean and prevent arteriosclerosis.

Three recent studies clearly show the deadly effects of trans-fats. More than 85,000 women were studied for eight years by Harvard Medical School. They tracked trans-fat intake and heart disease. The women with the highest trans-fat intake had a 50% higher rate of heart attacks and coronary artery disease.

The Agricultural University in the Netherlands did a study that showed trans-fats increase cholesterol to the same degree as saturated fats. Three groups of men and women with normal cholesterol were studied. Their diets were identical except for the type of fat consumed: saturated, trans-fat and polyunsaturated. After 3 weeks the saturated and trans-fat groups had elevated cholesterol. Their LDL cholesterol (bad, artery clogging kind) rose while the 'good' HDL cholesterol fell. This didn't happen in the polyunsaturated group.

A German study demonstrated the ill affects on premature babies. The higher the level of trans-fats in the newborn's blood the lower the birth weight and chance of survival.

As mentioned before, trans-fats like lard are generally solid at body temperature, while cis-fats remain liquid at body temperature. This makes them more sticky and likely to clog our arteries. Our platelets and other blood cells are also more sticky because of the trans-fats that become incorporated in their membranes. Trans-fats also interfere with prostaglandin production and hence kidney function, protection against ulcers, blood pressure and immune system function. Trans-fats worsen an essential fatty acid (EFA) deficiency. They do this by clogging up the enzyme reactions that transform fatty acids into highly unsaturated fatty acid derivatives. These highly unsaturated fatty acids are necessary for normal function of the brain, sense organs, testes and adrenals.

Trans-fats are not found in the plant world; they do not occur in fruits, vegetables, nuts or seeds. Significant amounts of trans-fats, (about 15%) are found in dairy and animal products. The main sources of trans-fats are from margarine, shortening, animal products and any cooked fats and oils. Most supermarket breads, cookies, crackers, chips and packaged foods are loaded with partially hydrogenated oils, a big source of trans-fats. Trans-fats do not appear on labels and are not considered saturated fat so label reading becomes more difficult. Just remember to ***avoid all products with partially hydrogenated oils.*** The detrimental effects of trans-fats are so well documented that the Dutch government banned the sale of margarines containing trans-fats. The head of Harvard School of Medicine, Dr. Walter Willet, says that over 300,000 American lives are lost each year to heart disease just due to the harmful effects of margarine on the heart.

Some more effects of trans-fats include:

- Decreased testosterone and increase abnormal sperm (in animals).
- Interference with pregnancy.
- Associated with low birth weight babies.
- Decrease the quality of breast milk.
- Promotes diabetes.
- Decreases the livers ability to process toxins.
- Alter size, number and composition of human fat cells.
- Alter immune function.

We now know the detrimental effects of trans-fats on our cardiovascular system, immune system, reproductive system hormonal systems, metabolism, liver function and cell membranes.

So why would we ever consume any margarines, shortenings, partially hydrogenated oil or any refined oils?

AVERAGE TRANS-FAT COMPOSITION OF FOODS

(Number in parentheses shows the range)

MARGARINES	
Stick	31% (10-48%)
Tub	17% (5-44%)
"Low Fat"	(up to 18%)
BUTTER (Milk Fat)	15%
VEGETABLE SHORTENING	20% (up to 37%)
SALAD OILS	(0-14%)
FRENCH FRIES	(up to 37%)
CANDY BARS	(up to 39%)
BAKERY PRODUCTS	(up to 34%)

While trans-fats are definitely injurious to our well-being, healthy oils can also be turned into toxic oils by air, heat and light. Many of the oils available in stores are damaged by processing, particularly the healthiest oils because they are the most biologically active.

Frying and cooking with oils

High temperatures destroy the health promoting characteristics of biologically reactive oils. The more unsaturated and the higher the proportion of essential fatty acids (EFAs), the more unhealthy it becomes. Not only are deadly trans-fats created, but dozens of other oxidation products are made far more toxic than trans-fatty acids. Our bodies can cope with an occasional dose of a toxic substance. But over 10, 20, or 30 years these toxic and unnatural substances accumulate and interfere with the normal biological chemistry of our bodies. Cells will begin to degenerate leading to degenerative disease and rapid aging.

I do not recommend frying not only because of the fat damage but because it destroys much of the nutritional value of all food. Frying can also turn proteins into carcinogens such as acrolein. In Udo Erasmus's book *Fats that Heal, Fats that Kill,* he recommends using saturated fats to fry like tropical oils or high oleic oils. While saturated fats are very unhealthy, they are much less reactive and form fewer toxic fats when heated at high temperatures. Damage occurs rapidly to unsaturated fats and even more rapidly to essential fatty acids (EFAs). Most fast food and other restaurants deep fry foods in hydrogenated vegetable oils that have been kept at high temperatures for days. Oils kept at 215° C (419° F) for 15 minutes or more consistently produced atherosclerosis when fed to experimental animals.

Instead of frying, try traditional stirfry vegetables and steam them for a few minutes. Then add flax seed oil that has had garlic pressed into it and allow to marinate for about 15 minutes. Another "healthier" way of frying is to stirfry with small amounts of water adding the oil later. Keeping some water in with the oil keeps the temperature down to 100° C (212°F), a non-destructive temperature. Food will retain more nutrients and taste better using this method. Use organic Canola or virgin olive oil for this method. Organic oils are pesticide free and unrefined. Refining an oil takes away its natural flavors and many nutrients—phytosterol, lecithin, carotene, tocopherols and EFAs.

Boiling in water doesn't damage even the most sensitive EFA rich oils. Baking does damage sensitive oils on the outside of baked goods like the crust of bread. If you don't use non-stick pans use tropical oils to prevent sticking.

The more unsaturated or damaged oils you consume, the more antioxidants you need in your diet to neutralize the excess free radicals that are formed by these oils.

Polyunsaturated Oils Linked to Cancer

Consuming large amounts of *refined* polyunsaturated oils has been linked to cancer. The more unsaturated the fat the more likely it is to form free radicals. Free radicals are unstable molecules that can disrupt cellular functioning, encourage tumor formation and speed the aging process. Free radicals have also been implicated in damaging arterial walls. Damage to arterial walls and free radical oxidation of LDL cholesterol are probably the initiatory steps in arteriosclerosis and atheroma formation. The free radical causes an injury to the arterial wall and a oxidized cholesterol ladened plaque forms, like a bandage over the injury. If this happens often enough, arteries will close off causing strokes, heart attacks and vascular disease.

The body will slowly unclog these vessels if chronic damage by free radicals is stopped or slowed down. Free radicals oxidize cholesterol and triglycerides to a more deadly artery clogging form. Fortunately, free radicals can be neutralized by free radical scavengers (antioxidants) such as vitamin E, beta-carotene, vitamin C, selenium and hundreds of other antioxidants found in unrefined oils (especially low temperature, expeller pressed wheat germ oil), fresh vegetables, fruits, whole grains, legumes and raw nuts and seeds. **Animal products are high in free radicals and almost totally deficient in antioxidants.**

Rejuvenating Oils—Essential Fatty Acids

There are just two essential fatty acids *linoleic acid (LA) and alpha-linolenic acid (LNA)* . Sixty percent of the population gets too much LA while ninety-five percent gets too little LNA. LA is found in vegetable oils– safflower oil is 75% LA and sunflower oil is 65% LA. LA is absolutely required for optimal health; most people are not deficient in LA. LNA is also absolutely required for optimal health. LNA is also called an omega-3 fatty acid. Most American diets are sadly deficient in LNA. The best source is flax seed oil which is about 60% LNA, about 10 times higher than most other available nut or seed oils. Other significant sources of LNA include Canola oil at 10%, soybean oil at 5-7% and walnut oil at 3-11%,. Other common oils virtually have none. Most dark green leafy vegetables have very little oil, but this oil is 50% LNA.

Gamma-linoleic acid (GLA) is identical to LNA except for the position of one of its double bonds. Because of their similarity their health benefits are similar. GLA is a great supplement for a stressed body or anyone over 40. Our bodies don't always make enough GLA and people with liver problems, inflammatory diseases and premenstrual syndrome will experience tremendous benefits from GLA along with a sound nutritional program.[x]

Udo Erasmus recommends about 1 tablespoon of LA per day and about two thirds as much LNA. Supplement vegetarian diets[y] with 2-4 tablespoons of Omega organic flax seed meal and one borage capsule every day. Use flax seed oil and olive oil.

Flax Seed Oil

One of the best nutritional oils for reversing the degenerative process is flax seed oil. However, it is extremely sensitive to air, light and heat. There is only one company I know of that has done extensive research and gone to great expense to produce flax seed oil with minimal exposure to these damaging environmental agents. That company is Spectrum Naturals.

The Spectrum Naturals Response

It was the knowledge that extraordinary precautions were necessary to produce an oil rich in omega-3 fatty acids that

---

[x] More on GLA in a couple pages.

[y] If you eat significant amounts of meat or other bad oils then use 4 Tbs. ground flax.

inspired the Spectrum Naturals company to develop a revolutionary new oil extraction technology, the SpectraVac process. Spectrum Naturals uses this process to make Veg Omega-3 Organic Flax Oil and other nutritional supplement oils. This unique oil removal process eliminates the damaging consequences of light, air and heat.

Spectrum Naturals is the only processor to use in-line refrigeration between the seed press, oil storage and settling vessels (which are also refrigerated). This extra step provides the oil maximum protection from damaging heat. Other manufacturers refrigerate only at the store. Not only do Spectrum Naturals refrigerate after crushing, settling and filling, but they make every effort to ship their Veg Omega-3 by refrigerated truck and ensure that distributors and retailers properly care for the oil. No one can protect as well as Mother Nature, but in the SpectraVac process Spectrum takes every additional step they can to try to protect as well as Mother Nature. I know first-hand about this extraordinary process because I asked for a tour of their SpectraVac processing plant and was very impressed.

You can find Spectrum Naturals Veg Omega-3 Organic Flax Oil in the refrigerator section of your health food store. Make sure you keep it in your refrigerator and use it up within six weeks. I keep ours in the freezer as it remains a liquid.

I think Udo Erasmus said it best in his critique of fresh flax-seed oil in his book, *Fats and Oils*. "The fresh oil of the very useful flaxseed is the very best oil there is, in every way. It looks good: a rich, deep golden color like fresh liquid sunshine—which by the way, it is. The aroma is a gentle, pleasant, nutty bouquet. It has a variety of flavors. It varies depending on where it is grown to being robust and slightly bitter to light and nutty. Its texture is so light that it is hard to believe that it is oil at all. We usually associate oil with a 'heavy, oily' texture. Not so for flax."

I include it in blender drinks, in salad dressings, sprinkle it on steamed vegetables and potatoes. Use your imagination. Just don't heat it, keep it refrigerated, and use it up before the expiration date on the bottle.

Wheat Germ Oil

It contains 50% LA and is one of the richest sources of vitamin E, octacosanol, and beta sitosterin. Because of its highly reactive nature LA can form free radicals. Therefore, vitamin E is needed to protect us from this damaging process. The vitamin E in wheat germ oil is natural mixed tocopherols (d-alpha, beta and gamma) and not just d-alpha like most vitamin E capsules. Beta and gamma are also free radical scavengers that all work in harmony. Octacosanol is a 28-carbon fatty alcohol that is a potent source of energy prized by competitive athletes. It also protects heart function and may help in nerve regeneration. Beta sitosterin is a phytosterol that assists in the digestion of fats.

Borage, Black Currant and Evening Primrose Oils

These oils are the primary sources of GLA. These oils usually come in capsules and the oils are often contaminated with solvents used to extract the oil or pesticides used in growing the plant. I choose cold pressed organic oils. The only reason I take borage oil is because it has 24% GLA. Black currant contains up to 18% and evening primrose contains 9%.

Our bodies can make GLA from LA if conversion isn't blocked. Conversion of LA to GLA can be blocked by eating any of the unhealthy fats previously mentioned or refined vegetable oils. Dietary deficiencies, high sugar or alcohol consumption, viral infections, diabetes and just plain aging can also block conversion. Consuming GLA will bypass this blockage but that is not a reason to continue with an unhealthy diet.

Mediterranean Diet

In 1958, Ancel Keys and an international team of scientists set out to discover the causes of heart disease. The evidence at the time seemed to implicate fat as the major cause. Keys and his wife traveled Europe and Africa measuring cholesterol levels. Their most significant finding was that affluent people, who ate more meat and dairy, were more likely to suffer heart attacks and have high cholesterol than poor people.

Another piece of supportive evidence was the fact that during World War II heart disease plummeted in countries with shortages of meat and dairy products.

To further investigate diet's role in heart disease, Keys and his research team studied 12,000 healthy middle aged men from 7 countries for 20 years. He discovered that the highest incidence of heart disease (28%) was in Finland. The Finns ate 24% of their calories from saturated fat (mostly from dairy products).

The lowest rate of heart disease didn't go to the Japanese who had the lowest amount of fat in their diets (9% of their calories from fat and only 3% from saturated fat). The Japanese heart disease rate low at 5%, was not nearly as good as the 655 men studied from the Greek island of Crete. After 10 years only 2% developed heart disease and none of them had died.

Amazingly, the men from Crete ate about as much total fat as the Finns. Their saturated fat was 8%, almost twice that of the Japanese.

The Cretan diet was low in meat and dairy, it consisted of beans, fresh fruits and vegetables with over half of their calories coming from whole grain bread and olive oil.

Olive Oil

There has been a lot of press lately about the health benefits of olive oil. It seems to protect against heart disease and is associated with low cancer incidence and overall good health. Olive oil is high in monounsaturated and unsaturated fatty acids that protect our body's cells from mutation, that is if it is *virgin or extra virgin* olive oil. Virgin olive oils are the only *mass* marketed oils that have not been heated above 150° C (302° F). When oils are heated higher than this they not only lose their protective effects but they become damaging to the body. Refined oils are heated at much higher temperatures that creates mutated oils. Furthermore, in processing oils, they may use poisonous solvents to extract the oil left behind after pressing. They may degum the oils with phosphoric acid (an extremely caustic chemical) which removes several health promoting substances such as lecithin, chlorophyll and several minerals. The oils may then be bleached and deodorized with more chemicals and heats up to 270° C (518° F) for 30 to 60 minutes. Fully processed olive oil loses over 100 volatile compounds that gives olive oil its unique flavors and aromas. The final product of all this is a mutated oil stripped of all its healthy components including EFAs. The bottom line on buying healthy oils is to get, organically grown cold pressed oils that are protected from light, air and heat.

Another health benefit of olive oil is better blood sugar control. Four different medical centers studied 42 non-insulin dependent diabetics. Half of the group ate a diet with the traditional 55% of the calories from carbohydrates and 30% from fat. The other half ate only 40% of calories from carbohydrates and a whopping 45% from fat, with highly monounsaturated olive oil as the predominant fat.

The low-carb, high-mono diet resulted in better diabetic control—lower day long blood levels of glucose, insulin and triglycerides. These benefits persisted throughout the 14 week study. Cholesterol and blood lipid levels were not increased.

In his book *Sunlight*, Zane Kime, M.D. espouses the benefits of sunlight in preventing cancer and promoting health. He claims skin cancer is promoted by a poor diet, particularly refined fats, oils and animal products. Recent research has tied skin cancer to a diet too high in omega-6 fatty acids and deficient in omega-3 fatty acids.

Another medical doctor, Dr. Edward N. Siguel, M.D., Ph.D, has written a book, *Essential Fatty Acids in Health and Disease*. Dr. Siguel writes that cardiovascular disease and cancer can be prevented in many cases by controlling the balance of EFAs in our diet.

Hundreds of studies have shown the disease producing effects of animal fats, trans-fats and too much omega-6 fatty acids. Research has also demonstrated the disease fighting effects of the omega-3 fatty acids. Now you have more knowledge to improve your health. The choice is yours.

Flaxseed: Nature's Miracle Medicine

Nothing But the Flax!

Often referred to as "nutritional gold," flaxseed is a wonder grain of health. It can heal and prevent cardiovascular disease, cancer, diabetes and many other degenerative conditions associated with aging. When my patients have problems with dry skin I prescribe ground flaxseed. Side benefits include healthy hair, bowels and many more.

For more than fifty centuries, flaxseed (also known industrially as linseed) has been consumed by humankind. The main foods mentioned in the Bible are flax, wheat, barley, corn, wine and manna—flax being referred to most often. It is one of the oldest known cultivated plants. According to archaeological authorities on the subject, in 5000 BC flax was being cultivated in Babylon. The ancient Egyptians used it to make linen mummy wrappings around 3000 BC. The Greek and Roman writings dating 650 BC reveal some of the healing properties of flax. In the 5th century BC, Hippocrates wrote about using flax to relieve inflamed mucous membranes and for relieving abdominal pains and diarrhea. History also points to flax being used in hot compresses to treat both external and internal ailments. Some of the ancient East Indian scriptures state that a yogi must eat flax daily in order to reach the highest state of contentment and joy.

> *"Whenever flaxseed becomes a regular food item among the people, there will be better health."*
> —Mahatma Gandhi

In Vedic lore, flax is considered a "cooling" oil—reducing inflammation.

In the past you were more likely to find flax derivatives in your house paint, linoleum floor, and bed linens than on your plate.

Times are changing. Today edible flaxseed is being rediscovered by people who are health oriented. Before long, flaxseed and its healing oil may be hailed as the latest in the fight against cancer and coronary heart disease, according to plant biochemists and researchers.

What makes this plant so beneficial? During the last decade research scientists have uncovered components of the flaxseed which offer greater physiological advantages than most other foods.

A real powerhouse, this seed packs a quadruple whammy:
1. High dose of omega-3 fatty acids, a healthy fat which helps lower cholesterol.[z]
2. Potent source of vitamins, minerals and protein.
3. Fiber, especially cholesterol lowering soluble fiber.
4. Lignans, a kind of fiber that is looking more and more like a potent blocker of some kinds of cancer.

All this, and it tastes good, too. It's hard to believe that flax is full of fat and still good for you.

Let's look more closely at flax and its highly regarded nutritional components. Flax is an annual plant with small green leaves and delicate blue flowers. Its Latin name is Linum Usitatissimum, meaning "the most useful." This miracle grain is truly one of the most nutritionally complete foods ever studied.

Flaxseed is a top quality food because it contains most of what makes a complete diet. According to Udo Erasmus in his book *Fats that Heal, Fats that Kill*, the components of flax are used to treat many ailments which wouldn't occur if flaxseed were a regular part of the diet.

Flax seed is a healthy source of:
Protein—Flaxseeds contain high quality, easily digestible protein that contains all amino acids (the building blocks of protein)

---

[z] See the chapter: Deadly Fats vs. Healing Fats.

essential to human health. This means that it is a complete protein. These essential amino acids are leucine, isoleucine, lysine, valine, threonine, methionine, phenylalanine and tryptophan. Flaxseed also contains histidine and arginine which are amino acids essential for infants. When all of the essential amino acids are supplied, our body can manufacture from them the other dozen amino acids required to make proteins. Complete proteins are essential for building our muscles, blood, skin, hair, nails and internal organs, including the heart and the brain.

Complex Carbohydrates—Flaxseed provides instant calories for energy and assist in digestion and regulation of protein and fat metabolism.

Fiber—Flaxseed is an excellent source of both soluble and insoluble fiber and keeps the digestive tract from becoming clogged with mucus. Fiber helps to keep everything moving, maintains healthy intestinal flora and helps to keep the colon clean. It also helps to keep cholesterol and bile acids from being re-absorbed into the body though the intestinal walls.

Mucilage—It is a thick gum found in many plants, especially flax seed (12%-15%) which makes the venerable flaxseed one of the best natural laxatives available. Like the pectin found in apples, mucilage in flax is important to bowel regularity. It soothes and protects the delicate stomach and intestinal linings and keeps the contents moving smoothly along. One of the most highly respected natural healers, Bernard Jensen, reveals that many degenerative diseases start in our colon through the toxic effects of constipation. When flaxseed is taken with fluids, the mucilage assists in alleviating constipation, increasing stool bulk and softness, and speeding up transit time (hastens the movement of stool out of our body). All this helps prevent toxic buildup in our bowel. As a result, the stools smell less foul, our breath freshens, and there is less stress on our eliminative organs including the liver, kidneys, and skin. Flax mucilage also has the ability to buffer excess acid in sensitive stomachs and helps to stabilize blood glucose.

Minerals—Flaxseed contains most known major and trace minerals—phosphorous, magnesium, potassium, calcium, sulfur, sodium, chlorine, zinc, iron and adequate trace amounts of manganese, silicon, copper, fluorine, nickel, cobalt, iodine, molybdenum and chromium.[aa]

Vitamins—Flaxseed contains fat-soluble vitamins E and carotene, and water-soluble vitamins B1, B2 and C. The tocopherols compounds found in vitamin E act as antioxidants in the body, protecting other molecules and cell components from damaging reactions with oxygen.

Lignins and Lignans—Unlike many other plant fibers, flax seed is high in *lignan* and *lignin*. Lignin is an insoluble fiber which our bodies convert to several kinds of *lignans*. Flaxseed is also the richest known source of lignans. Lignans have only recently attracted the attention of researchers. They have been found to be useful in treating viral, bacterial and fungal infections as well as cancer. In fact, high levels of lignans in the bowel are associated with reduced rates of colon and breast cancer. Flax contains 100 times the quantity of lignans as the next best source—wheat bran. In other words, while all vegetables provide lignan precursors to some degree, flax provides more, about 800 milligrams per gram, as compared to only eight milligrams per gram in common fiber such as bran.

The lignans formed from flax are "pseudo estrogens" that block estrogen receptors in the body. A potent cancer causing hormone, estrogen can, when over produced, stimulate colon cancer. 30 to 50 percent of all malignant colon tumors contain prodigious estrogen receptors. It is also significant to note that the rates of colon cancer tend to correlate with those of breast cancer, and that both seem to be high in people with low fiber diets. Studies reveal that lignans resemble estrogens and attach to estrogen receptors in the body, but do not have the tumor stimulating effect of hormonal estrogen. Further, research shows that lignans derived from flax also work to

---

[aa] See the chapter: Minerals.

reduce levels of unbound estrogens in the blood, which explains how they can also help prevent breast cancer. Perhaps the presence of lignans, derived from plant fiber, may be one of the main reasons why vegetarians have substantially lower cancer rates than meat eaters do.

Essential Fatty Acids—The essential fatty acids (EFAs) are part of every cell in our bodies, where they play important roles in maintaining the structure of the cells and in producing energy. Our glands need EFAs to carry out the minute secretion of hormones and other biological regulating substances. In our muscles, EFAs help the cells to recover from use and abuse. In addition to fulfilling these basic roles, the EFAs are critical to infants' prenatal and postnatal development, especially brain development, and for growth spurts throughout childhood.

Our bodies do a remarkable job of creating most of the nutrients we need from the resident cell materials on hand. Except in some cases. The nutrients our bodies can't synthesize are called the essential nutrients, and these we must make sure are adequately supplied in our diets. Of the 50 essential nutrients,[bb] three are fatty acids: called omega-3 (alpha-linolenic acid), gamma-linoleic acid and omega-6 (linoleic acid). Besides being an excellent source of the essential omega-3 fatty acids, flaxseed also contains important trace nutrients such as phospholipids, phytosterols, and beta-sistosterin. These naturally occurring compounds assist in the digestion of fats and are just beginning to be recognized for their immune enhancing properties.

The Modern Diet and Omega-3 Deficiency

In the past 100 years, modern food processing developments have drastically reduced the nutrient value, including the omega-3 content, of many of the foods we eat. Processing and refining is usually done to stabilize the foods and increase the shelf life or to change the texture of these food products. In his book *The Omega-*

[bb] See the chapter: Why Supplements?

3 Phenomenon, Dr. Donald O. Rudin explains that modern food processing and food selection opportunities severely distort the availability of many essential nutrients—especially limiting the omega-3 essential fatty acids. This is attributed to the use of high heat, sterilization and addition of caustic agents in the food. Whenever this occurs, the incidence of 20th century diseases skyrockets. Heart disease and many cancers finally are being recognized as being linked to distortions of dietary fats. Rudin calls omega-3 EFA "the nutritional missing link" and attributes its profound absence in most foods to the cause of many degenerative conditions.

For our bodily functions to stay healthy, we must have a proper balance of omega-3/omega-6 fatty acids in our diets. For example, when your body is homeostatic (balanced in health), pain messages come on only when you've experienced real injury or blood clots form as the initiating phase of wound healing. Without such homeostatic balance, the omega-6s (when consumed to excess and in absence of omega-3 EFA) can produce pain messages in the brain for no reason or form an unwanted clot spontaneously.

Most Americans who eat highly refined and processed diets, such as the regular patrons of fast food restaurants, get excess amounts of omega-6 and insufficient amounts of omega-3 fatty acids. The hamburger cooks and fish fryers of fast food restaurants usually cook with highly refined, unstable polyunsaturated oils such as corn, sunflower, safflower and soy oils. These oils are very highly concentrated with omega-6 fatty acids and health-destroying trans-fats due to excessive processing. Studies have shown trans-fats to be worse than saturated fat for health. The physiology of "fast food consumers" remains in a perpetual state of fatty acid imbalance. Consequently, they are more predisposed to degenerative processes such as heart attacks, cancer, arthritis, stroke, kidney impairment, liver disease, autoimmune disorders and dermal disorders.

According to Udo Erasmus, a highly regarded lipid (fat) scientist, we North Americans typically consume only about 25% of the quantity of omega-3s we need for optimal health. He suggests an intake of omega-3s equivalent to about 2% of total calories, or about 14 grams per day. ***Flaxseed is the most potent natural source of omega-3s.***

Fish oils have been touted for their "heart saving" omega-3 fatty acids found in the flesh of deep sea fatty fish, such as salmon and mackerel. But what are these animals doing with so much plant essential fatty acids in their fat? They obtain them from the algae and plankton that comprise the foundation of the ocean's food chain. But, unfortunately at the same time, research shows that the marine oils in these fish also contain traces of pesticides, heavy metals and other industrial pollutants, such as PCBs. According to Ralph Nader and other respected environmental activists, even our deep sea waters are now polluted, and the fish store the pollutants in their liver and fatty tissue. Organic flaxseed, fortunately, contains no such toxic residues.

Comparison of Omega-3 Sources

Percentage of Omega-3 Fatty Acid by Total Weight of Seeds

Flaxseed	**57%**
Chia Seed	**30%**
Hemp Seed Oil	**15%**
Pumpkin Seed	**15%**
Canola Oil	**10%**
Soy Bean Oil	**8%**
Walnut	**5%**
Fresh Leafy Vegetable (Average Serving)	**0.009%**

Omega-3s and the Health Connection

In the last ten years a plethora of scientific studies have been conducted on flaxseed and its nutritional oil. At a recent conference held at the Flax Institute of the United States in Fargo, ND, scientists focused attention on flaxseed and its role in healing and preventing numerous degenerative diseases. In fact, it was reported that omega-3 deficiencies contribute to many conditions and may be the ultimate cause of many wide spread degenerative diseases. A report from Health and Welfare Canada (comparable to our Food & Drug Administration) dispelled any fears about flaxseed's possible toxicity.

Research and clinical experience show that omega-3s have beneficial effects in:

1. **Cancers.** The National Cancer Institute is currently researching flaxseed for its potential ability to prevent cancer. Flaxseed is considered unique because of its abundant amount of lignan fiber and LNA (omega-3). And according to Dr. James Duke of the USDA (via the Data Base at the University of Illinois), flaxseed contains 27 identifiable cancer preventive compounds. As mentioned above, research evidence suggests that lignans may fight off chemicals responsible for initiating tumors and block estrogen receptors, which may reduce colon cancer risk.

   For over thirty-five years, German lipid researcher Johanna Budwig has been using flaxseed oil successfully in cancer therapy. She has more than 1,000 documented cases of successful cancer treatment with flaxseed oil as the main treatment. In his New York City clinic, the now deceased Max Gerson, M.D., used fresh flaxseed oil as the principle cancer fighting agent. More recent research show that **omega-3s kill human cancer cells in tissue culture without harming the normal cells present.** Breast, lung and prostate cancer cell lines were studied.

2. **Heart Disease.** Omega-3s lower high blood cholesterol and triglyceride levels from 25% to 65%. Dr. Gerson used fresh flaxseed oil for its cholesterol lowering ability. At the Department of Clinical Chemistry in Denmark, H. O. Bang discovered that Greenland Eskimos who consumed high omega-3 diets had only three cases of heart trouble among a population of 2,400 people over four years' study. Two of those cases were over 78 years old, and the other case was complicated with rheumatic fever.

It's interesting to us that some studies have suggested that high fat intake is a risk factor in cancer incidence, but Greenland Eskimos have a high total fat intake and relatively low rates of cancer. They also have a very low incidence of ischemic heart disease (the leading cause of death in the industrialized world), attributed to their diet which contains high levels of omega-3. This suggests that the prevention of cancer and heart disease is less related to the *quantity* of dietary fat and more related to the *quality* of fat we eat. Further studies showed that when Greenland Eskimos moved to Denmark and adopted the saturated fat Danish diet, they experience a higher heart attack rate, even though the total caloric fat content of their diet decreased. It was concluded that a relative deficiency of essential fatty acids is common in western diets and it plays an important part in the causation of atherosclerosis, diabetes, hypertension, and certain forms of malignant diseases.

It was further revealed that Eskimos' levels of total cholesterol and 'bad' LDL cholesterol were significantly lower and their levels of 'good' HDL cholesterol were higher than among Danes in all age groups and both sexes. In other words, even though the Eskimos' diet was higher in fat, their intake of omega-3 was much higher and their blood lipid (fat) levels were healthier.

One of the unique features of flaxseed is that it contains a substance which resembles the prostaglandins, which may well be part of its potent therapeutic value. Prostagladins regulate blood pressure and arterial function, and have an important role in calcium and energy metabolism. No other vegetable oil examined so far can match this property of flaxseed oil.

3. **Diabetes.** One form of this disease originates from a deficiency of omega-3s and an excess of hard fats. A concurrent lack of vitamins and minerals makes the disease worse. Omega-3s may also lower the insulin requirement of diabetics.

4. **Inflammatory Tissue Conditions.** The omega-3 fatty acid decreases inflammatory conditions of all types. These are the diseases that end in -itis, which include bursitis, tendinitis, tonsillitis, gastritis, ileitis, colitis, meningitis, arthritis, phlebitis, prostatitis, nephritis, splenitis, hepatitis, pancreatitis, otitis, etc. as will as lupus. Many of these inflammatory conditions may be eased by use of omega-3s.

5. **Skin Conditions.** Pedigree show animals are fed linseed oil, made from flaxseed, to keep their coats glossy. Along the same lines, recent research has shown that skin conditions in humans, such as psoriasis and eczema, have improved dramatically when flaxseed and flax oil was added to the diet. These skin conditions exacerbate from lack of omega-3s in the diet. You will see that your skin gets smoother, softer and velvety from taking flaxseed oil regularly. It's also helpful for treating dry skin, dandruff, and sun sensitive skin.

6. **Sexual Disorders.** Dr. Budwig has found flaxseed oil to be a nutritional aphrodisiac. The most common physical cause of impotency in men and non orgasmic response in women is blockage of blood flow in the arteries of the pelvis. Decrease of blood flow prevents full expansion (erection) of the penis and/or the clitoris. Thus ejaculation and/or orgasm cannot occur. The solution is to unblock narrowed arteries in general, and the consumption of flaxseed oil will aid one's body in doing that. The omega-3 components of flaxseed oil are known to prevent spontaneous blood clotting caused by an excess of Omega-6

fatty acids. Flaxseed oil is quickly gaining the reputation as one of the best aphrodisiacs of the 90s.

7. **Calmness Under Stress.** Many people find this to be the most profound effect of using fresh flaxseed oil. It brings on a feeling of calmness often within a few hours. This may be partly due to that fact that under stress, omega-3 fatty acids appear to slow down our bodies' production of toxic biochemicals.

Selye's "flight or fight syndrome" as a stress response is mitigated because the omega-3's compete against the arachadonic acid cascade which happens when we are stressed. Arachidonic acid in our blood thickens the blood platelets in anticipation of wounding and bleeding which is an ancient natural defense mechanism.

8. **Water Retention.** EFA's in flax oil helps the kidneys excrete sodium and water. Water retention (edema) accompanies swollen ankles, some forms of obesity, PMS and all stages of cancer and cardiovascular disease.

9. **Vitality and Athletic Ability.** One of the most noticeable signs of improved health from the use of flaxseed oil is the progressive and increased vitality and more energy. Athletes notice that their fatigued muscles recover from exercise more quickly. Omega-3's also increase stamina. According to East Indian Vedic medicine, flax generates a healing heat in the body. In simple terms, flax increases metabolic rate and the efficiency of cellular energy production. It stimulates respiratory and cellular oxidation by which energy is produced and we experience this as a sensation of warmth. For athletes, or anyone wishing to reduce fat and create a fit, lean body, this is great news! Finally, a healthy fat that doesn't make you fat. Adding flaxseed to the diet will enhance all life processes, because all our life processes depend on energy production.

10. **Other Conditions.** Omega-3s are necessary for visual function (retina), adrenal function (stress), and sperm formation. It often

improves symptoms of multiple sclerosis. In fact, when omega-3 consumption is high, MS is rare. Flax oil can also be helpful in cystic fibrosis (omega-3 containing oils help loosen viscous secretions and relieve breathing difficulties); some cases of sterility and miscarriage; some glandular malfunctions; some behavioral problems (schizophrenia, depression, bipolar disorder); allergies; addictions (to drugs or alcohol) and some addictive behaviors.

Fortified Flax Meal

Another beneficial way to get Omega-3s into your diet is by eating Fortified Flax. Keep in mind that if you swallow flaxseeds whole, your body will not get the nutrients they contain, because they are protected by a tough seed coat. In fact, after the seeds go through you, you could actually plant them and they would still grow. To break the seed coat and make the nutrients available for digestion, you can either grind the flaxseeds yourself or, better yet, get Fortified Flax in your health food store.

Fortified Flax, from the Omega-Life company, is a whole unrefined organic flaxseed that is fortified and stabilized in a unique grinding process. It is ground to release the many nutrients which are otherwise isolated by this protective seed hull. Vitamins and minerals are added to the product to keep it fresher and to help in the digestion and assimilation of nutrients. Its fortified with zinc, iron, niacin (B3), B6 and B12. This meal thus provides a food for humans that has all of the advantages of flaxseed discussed here and none of the disadvantages, like quick rancidity and free radical or trans-fatty acid formation when light, heat and air are not excluded. Fortified Flax is sealed in an oxygen barrier liner so no refrigeration is necessary until opening (you may refrigerate or freeze it before opening to extend its freshness).

In a study conducted under the care of Milwaukee Wellness Clinic, it was found that in only three weeks of taking 2 T. daily of Fortified Flax, serum triglyceride levels dropped almost 50% in subjects with above normal levels. Further research also shows that the use of freshly ground flaxseeds can also improve digestion, prevent and reverse constipation, stabilize blood glucose levels, improve cardiovascular health, inhibit tumor formation and bring about other benefits.

Make sure you take this ground flaxseed with plenty of fluid, because its mucilage absorbs 5 times the seeds weight of water. In addition to Spectrum Naturals Flax Oil, try from 1 to 2 tablespoons of Fortified Flax per day. Mix it in juice or water, blend it (see recipes), or sprinkle it on cereal, soups, salads and cooked grains.

Nature has provided us with everything we need to be healthy and free from disease. This is especially true when it comes to this marvelous plant the flax. Our ancestors knew instinctively that flax was nourishing, soothing and healing. Fortunately, their intuitive wisdom is now being confirmed by modern scientific analysis. The verdict is in: Everyone who studies it believes that flaxseed will continue to make great breakthroughs in the prevention and alleviation of disease. It's so easy to work it into your diet with Spectrum Veg Omega-3 Organic Flax Seed Oil and Fortified Flax, both available at your local health food store.

TOFU:
SUPERFOOD OR MIRACLE MEDICINE?

What if I told you there is a natural food that offers the following health benefits?

- It can help prevent ulcers by neutralizing stomach acid.
- It can help prevent breast and prostate cancer.
- It can mimic estrogen's positive effects on the skeletal, reproductive and cardiovascular system while blocking estrogen's carcinogenic effects on breast tissue.
- It decreases LDL cholesterol and in many ways helps prevent heart disease.
- It is a good source of calcium and prevents osteoporosis in several different ways.

There's more. It's inexpensive, readily available and easy to add to all of your favorite recipes. You'd probably want to rush out and buy a case of it. Right? What is this incredible product? It's tofu, made from soybeans. This little known product has been referred to as a 'superfood' or 'miracle medicine.'

Your are probably aware that the two greatest causes of death in America are heart disease and cancer. For years medical research has been looking for "the magic bullet" to prevent or cure these maladies. The pharmaceutical companies have developed several drugs that lower cholesterol. Unfortunately, in a number of these drug trials the overall death rate was unchanged or increased. Researchers in the United Kingdom and Finland reviewed these pharmaceutical studies and reported their results in the *British Medical Journal.* They concluded: **1) The death rate only increased in those trials using drugs to lower cholesterol.** 2)

Drug use should be halted except in severe cases until more research is done. 3) Dietary changes should be emphasized since they are safe and effective.

Scientific studies from all over the world reveals that **tofu and other soy products help prevent heart disease, cancer and other ailments as well.**

The Health Benefits of Soy Products—On February 20–23, 1994 in Mesa, Arizona, a number of research papers were presented at the *First International Symposium on the Role of Soy in Preventing and Treating Chronic Disease.* The presenters described the health benefits of soy. In this three-day conference doctors and respected researchers from around the world presented their work proving that soy helps to prevent disease. Although all the details are not yet known, we do know about many health promoting compounds. One of these is the isoflavone called *genistein.*

More than 200 studies have been published on genistein and many on its anti-cancer properties. Genistein works in much the same way as estrogen. It functions both as an estrogen agonist and antagonist; that is, it seems to promote the positive actions of estrogen while preventing many of its bad effects. It competitively binds to both estrogen receptors and progesterone receptors. These receptors are essential for tumor evolution and growth.

Kenneth Setchell of Children's Hospital Medical Center in Cincinnati, Ohio reports that dietary estrogens like genistein may play an important role in preventing hormone dependent diseases. He writes, "Recent studies of normally ovulating premenopausal women have shown that the dietary inclusion of soy protein (60g/day) specifically containing isoflavones leads to significant changes in the menstrual cycle, with the prolongation of cycle length, an increase in follicular phase length and a marked suppression of the mid cycle surge of gonadotrophins—luteinizing hormone and follicle-stimulating hormone." He added that these physiological effects would appear to decrease the risks of breast cancer.

Genistein seems to mimic Tamoxifen, the drug most commonly used to prevent recurrence of breast cancer. Genistein also resembles the drug Premarin in that it helps maintain trabecular bone decreasing the risk of osteoporosis. Studies reveal that soy products play an active role in the **prevention of osteoporosis** because they are a good source of the minerals boron and calcium. A 1988 study by the University of Texas Sciences Center showed that **volunteers excreted 50% less calcium in their urine when they replaced the animal products in their diets with soy foods.** Another way **genistein acts like Premarin is in reducing the terrible side effects of menopause.** According to a recent study in the respected British medical journal *Lancet*, eating tofu may reduce the frequency and severity of hot flashes.

A 1990 study at the Guy's Hospital in London found soy protein much easier on the kidneys than meat, which may be important for people with kidney disease.

Tofu Helps Fight Cancer—There are several compounds in soy products that help fight cancer. Genistein inhibits angiogenesis (the formation of new blood vessels) which is necessary for a rapidly growing tumor to feed itself. Saponins are naturally occurring compounds in soy beans, other legumes and some other foods. Saponins significantly reduced the growth and viability of cancerous colon cells and melanoma cells invitro, according to A. Venket Rao of the University of Toronto in Canada.

Another study of 8,000 Hawaiian men with Japanese ancestry published in *Cancer Research* in 1989 found that **men who ate the most tofu had the lowest rates of prostate cancer,** with other influences factored out. Similarly, a study in Singapore reported in the *Lancet (1991)* found that premenopausal females who rarely ate soy foods had twice the risk of breast cancer than those who ate soy foods frequently. All other food and lifestyle differences were taken into account. In both of these cases it was the *soy alone which made the difference, not the amount of fat.*

Cancer formation is actually a long process. The time span between tumor initiation and outright malignancy generally takes decades. There is a considerable time frame wherein the carcinogenic process could be halted or reversed through various chemopreventative strategies. We have already discussed many compounds in soy that inhibit or reverse cancer. Protease inhibitors are also potent anticarcinogens both in the body and in the test tube. A specific protease inhibitor derived from soybeans is Bowman-Birk inhibitor (BBI). BBI has been shown to suppress carcinogenesis; 1) in three different species; 2) several organ systems; 3) in different cell types; 4) different types of cancer; 5) by dietary inclusion as well as injection. Phytic acid and lignans are other compounds found in soy products that play a powerful role in cancer prevention.

The Role of Soy Protein in Reducing Heart Disease—Soy protein decreases LDL cholesterol and is effective in suppressing peroxidized LDL formation (this is the worst form of LDL cholesterol, a major contributor to atheroma formation).

Soy protein was also shown to consistently elevate plasma thyroxin concentrations in laboratory animals. Thyroxin is the primary hormone regulating metabolism. Increasing thyroxin will speed the metabolism, burn fat and decrease cholesterol. For those of you who are interested in having a fit, lean body, this is great news!

At the University of Milan's Center for the Study of Metabolic Diseases and Hyperlipidemia, Cesare Sirtori, M.D. studied the cholesterol lowering effects of adding soy protein to a low fat diet. One group of volunteers were fed soy protein while the control group remained on a low fat diet. Within two weeks, the serum cholesterol of the subjects eating soy foods dropped an average of

14%; in four weeks it dropped about 21%. The control subjects still on a low fat diet had no drop in cholesterol levels. Some of the soy eating group were asked to discontinue soy while maintaining their low fat diet. Their cholesterol levels crept back up to their previous levels in just two weeks. His conclusion was that soy alone was responsible for the decreased cholesterol levels.

To challenge the results of the first study, a group of volunteers was given a supplement of cholesterol (500mg/day) to see if that would negate the effects of soy. Despite the added cholesterol, these volunteers experienced the same drop in cholesterol as those who were given no cholesterol supplements.

More than 25 studies that have shown **substituting soy for animals protein or simply adding soy protein to the diet significantly reduces cholesterol, regardless of the type of fat in the diet.**

In the October 1993 *American Journal of Clinical Nutrition*, John Potter, M.D. reports that volunteers with only moderately high cholesterol levels (about 240mg./dl) experienced a 12% decrease in cholesterol levels in 4 weeks. This was accomplished by eating muffins made with 50mg. of soy protein each day. In a second trial the soy protein was cut in half to 25mg. per day and still the people with moderate to high cholesterol had a significant drop.

"The more soy people eat, the better, but even moderate amounts have an effect," says Potter. By moderate amounts he is referring to a couple of servings of soy foods each day such as a container of tofu in a stirfry and/or blender drink each day.

Protein: Tofu vs. Meat—Many people consider chicken a healthy protein source. I don't, three and one half ounces of white chicken meat contains 11 grams of fat and more than 3 of these are saturated fat. (It's also fraught with chemicals added to the chickens' food and has the potential to cause Salmonella poisoning). You can eat three times as much tofu, get as much quality protein (about 25 grams) with half the fat and 42 fewer calories. Also tofu has no cholesterol and its natural oils from soy are full of healthy essential fatty acids usually deficient in the Standard American Diet (SAD). An even better choice is now available called "Lite" tofu from Mori-Nu. It has only 35 calories in each 3 ounce serving and only 0.7 grams of fat. It's the only low fat tofu on the market.

Meats, including chicken have been implicated as the primary cause of heart disease. According to Dean Ornish, M.D. in his book *Eat More Weigh Less*, meat gives you a quadruple whammy.

Meat is:

- High in cholesterol, which clogs up all your arteries including your heart.
- High in saturated fat, which raises your blood cholesterol level.
- High in oxidants, like iron, which oxidize cholesterol to a form that is more easily deposited in your arteries.
- Low in healthy antioxidants.

In contrast, tofu and other forms of soy products give you more than a quadruple benefit.

Tofu:

- Contains no cholesterol.
- Contains no saturated fat.
- Has no free radicals (oxidants).
- Is high in naturally occurring antioxidants.
- Increases the uptake and degradation of LDL "bad" cholesterol.

How is Tofu Made?—Regular tofu is similar to cheese in its processing. While cheese is made from animal milk, tofu is made from soy milk. Soy milk is made from crushed soybeans and water.

Tofu is then made by coagulating the soy milk with a salt such as calcium chloride or an acid like lemon juice. The soy protein is transformed into curds and whey. The liquid whey is removed and the curds are pressed into blocks of tofu. Similarly in the manufacture of cheese, the best proteins are discarded with the whey, leaving a poorer quality protein known as casein.

Fortunately, a new revolutionary process of tofu production, developed by Morinaga, coagulates fresh soy milk right in the box. This preserves the whey and produces a smooth "silken style" tofu. The aseptic[cc] packaging requires no refrigeration until opened. Preserving the whey may hold on to some essential health promoters normally lost in the standard tofu manufacture. The aseptic process increases nutrient retention and flavor while ensuring safety. According to the Institute of Food Technologists, aseptic packaging is the most significant food science innovation of the last half-century.

Tofu is "Recipe Friendly"—I used to put up with the old fashioned tofu because I was aware of its health benefits. It was a hassle to deal with, because the tofu was bathed in water. We had to change it every day and it often spilled. To make matters worse, it was high in fat, even though it was "good" fat. Over 50% of its calories came from fat.

I now only use "Lite" tofu in aseptic packages. My favorite way to add tofu to our diet is in blender drinks with fresh or frozen fruit. The great thing about tofu is that it will take on any flavor. You can marinate it and make shish-ka-bobs, make dips and pates or add it to anything you are cooking, from pasta to vegetable dishes.[dd]

See the references in the back of the book.

[cc] Aseptic—no bacteria are present.

[dd] See the recipe chapter for recipes with for more free recipes, including an unbelievable low-fat chocolate dream pie, call: 1-800-NOW-TOFU.

WHY SHOULD WE TAKE SUPPLEMENTS?

As a doctor one of the most-asked questions I hear are: "Is it important to take nutritional supplements and which ones do I take and recommend?" This is how I usually answer these questions.

It would be great if we never needed to take supplements. 50 years ago, it was possible to be healthy simply by eating wholesome foods and living a wellness lifestyle. Very few of us today live a balanced lifestyle—eating home grown vital foods, breathing clean air, drinking fresh, non-contaminated water, exercising regularly and living stress-free. Wouldn't that be terrific?

Living our high-demand lifestyle, places extra requirements on our bodys. We need the additional support and protection that supplementation gives us. Even with a healthy, plant-based diet, emphasizing fresh fruits, vegetables, whole grains and legumes, the depletion of soil minerals leaves a void that must be filled. Further, an additional stress may be placed on our bodies by pollutants and radiation exposure.

If you smoke, drink alcohol or take medications, you need the extra protection that good supplements give you. Even when you exercise, your body creates harmful free radicals which can be neutralized by taking antioxidants.

Without a doubt, with all the changes and stresses in our lives, we need all the help we can get—and nutritional support is an important ally.

To build a healthy body it takes over 50 essential nutrients:
- 3 essential fatty acids.
- 8 essential amino acids (more for children).
- 13-16 vitamins.
- 20 or 21 minerals (we're not sure yet about tin).
- 40 more minerals for optimal health.

- A source of energy (carbohydrates are the cleanest source).
- Fiber (both soluble and insoluble).
- Bacteria (acidophilus, bifidus, streptofaecium and more).
- Enzymes (supplements may be neccessary in disease or poor dietary habits).
- Water.
- Oxygen.
- Light.

Almost all disease[ee] is caused by a deficiency of one or more of these 50 factors. I have never had a patient that didn't improve their health by getting these in their diet. Disease results from loss of health. Chemically, we need optimum amounts of these 50 nutrients. We also need to minimize our exposure to toxins.

Accessory nutrients—In addition to 50 essential factors, there are accessory nutrients which may be essential because of one of the following conditions: aging, disease, allergies, infection, injury, obesity, years of suboptimal nutrition or a genetic individuality. Some of the accessory nutrients include non-essential amino acids, carnitine, orotic acid, pangamic acid, coenzyme Q10, inosine, choline, inositol, lipoic acid, para-amino-benzoic acid (PABA), N-acetyl glucosamine (NAG), N-acetyl cysteine (NAC), hormones and neurotransmitters derived from amino acids, EFA derivatives and bioflavonoids. There are also thousands of health promoting substances in whole foods and herbs.

Standard American Diet (SAD)—has created deficiency disease in this country. Udo Erasmas reports in his book *Fats that Heal, Fats that Kill*, that—"Two government surveys, known as the Health and Nutrition Examination Survey (HANES, 1971-1974) and the Nationwide Food Consumption Survey (NFCS, 1977-1978), measured intake of 13 of about 50 essential nutrients in

---

[ee] Except that caused by genetic, emotional or spiritual sickness.

thousands of Americans. Of the 13, only sodium was present in adequate amounts (actually, many people suffer toxic symptoms from an excess of sodium resulting from the overuse of table salt). They found the following percentages of Americans getting less than the government-set Recommended Daily Allowance (RDA), which was defined as the amount of an essential nutrient that is sufficient to keep most normal healthy adults from developing deficiency symptoms."

Nutrient	% people who get less than RDA	Nutrient	% people who get less than RDA
Calcium	68%	Vitamin B_1	45%
Folacin	10+%	Vitamin B_2	34%
Iron	57%	Vitamin B_3	33%
Magnesium	75%	Vitamin B_6	80%
Phosphorus	27%	Vitamin B_{12}	34%
Vitamin A	50%	Vitamin C	41%

Clinicians and other experts 'unofficially' estimate the incidence of deficiency of other nutrients as:

Nutrient	% people who get less than RDA
Biotin	10%
Silicon	30%
Chromium	90%
Vitamin D	10%
Copper	85-90%
Vitamin E	20-40%
Manganese	20-30%
Vitamin K	15%
Pantothenic Acid	25%
Omega-3 FAs	95%
Selenium	50-60%
Zinc	35-60%

Major Source of Deficiencies—Food processing is the number one cause of nutrient deficiency—look what happens when whole wheat grain is turned into white flour:[ff]

Mineral	Loss (%)	Other Nutrient	Loss (%)
Calcium	60	Strontium	95
Chromium	40	Zinc	78
Cobalt	89	Vitamins B_1, B_2, & B_3	72-81
Copper	68	Vitamin B_6	72
Iron	76	Pantothenic Acid	50
Magnesium	85	Folic Acid	67
Manganese	86	Vitamin E	86
Molybdenum	48	Linoleic Acid	95
Phosphorus	71	Alpha-Linolenic Acid	95
Potassium	77	Protein	33
Selenium	16	Fiber	95

Similar loss is created in other grains including rice. Sugar has lost between 83-100% of each mineral present in raw sugar. The majority of calories in the Standard American Diet (SAD) come from depleted foods, 17% from sugar, 18% from refined grains & cereals, 3% from alcohol and 20% from refined fats. About 30% of the SAD diet comes from animal products, meat, milk and eggs. Animal products create more of a drain on our nutritional need than they contribute.

> **Only 11% of the Standard American Diet ☹**
> **comes from whole foods!**

Modern agriculture has robbed us of essential minerals—Depletion of our soils was discovered back in the 1950's—today studies have shown that North American soils have lost an average of 85% mineral content compared to 100 years ago. Large farms

---

[ff] The figures are from work done by Henry A. Schroeder in the U.S. and by M.O. Bruker in Germany, both MDs.

continually produce crops in the same soil year after year without replacing all the essential minerals. The agricultural industry only add what it has to produce their crop. The result is normal looking fruits and vegetables with drastically reduced mineral content. Fifty or more important minerals may be completely absent. Gabriel Cousen, M.D. reports the following in his book, *Conscious Eating*: "in the Firman Bear report on research done at Rutgers University, organically grown foods were much richer in minerals than the "look alike" commercial produce. For example, organic tomatoes had more than 5 times more calcium, 12 times more magnesium, 3 times more potassium, 68 times more manganese and 1,900 times more iron. The comparison of other produce was similar. **The overall estimate of the Rutgers research suggested that organic foods had 87% more minerals and trace elements than food that was commercially grown."**

Dr. Linus Pauling two time Nobel Laureate, once said, in his opinion one could **"trace every sickness, every disease and every ailment to a mineral deficiency."** Dr. Joel Wallach a veterinarian and naturopathic physician agrees.[gg]

Supplements—As you may be aware, supplementation is a huge business—over $4 billion a year market. And this is in part due to the recent acceptance of nutritional supplementation into mainstream medicine and the hundreds of new studies showing their efficacy in the treatment and prevention of disease. This has created a prolific growth of public use of supplements.

Just because a company makes supplements doesn't mean they are top quality. How do you know that supplements are true-to-label, genuine, high quality and made of the best forms of vitamins, minerals and other nutrients? The fact is you don't.

In a recent study, Linda Shaffer and Michelle Fairchild of Yale New Haven Hospital, evaluated 257 brands of vitamins purchased from pharmacies, grocery stores and health food stores. Many

---

[gg] See the chapter: Minerals.

were incomplete or had too little or too much of one or other nutrient. Only 49 were considered adequate.

Here are some guidelines to keep in mind when selecting the best supplements.

Good companies will put in the right amounts rather than token amounts of expensive compounds. Potencies are extremely important. What good does it do to take a herb that is so weak you would have to consume a pound of it to get what is needed? There are standardized potencies for most herbs, make sure you are getting what you pay for. Buying calcium can be confusing, make sure the label states the elemental quantities of minerals—the actual amount of the mineral element itself. For example, if a label for a calcium supplement reads: *2 tablets of calcium gluconate .... 1,000mg.*, you might think you're getting lots of calcium. Right? Calcium gluconate is only 9% elemental calcium which means 2 tablets contain only 90 mg of calcium, an insignificant amount. You'd have to take 26 of these pills to get the RDA! (Other common sources of calcium include calcium acetate (23% calcium), calcium citrate (21% calcium) and calcium lactate (14% calcium). For comparison, milk is less than 1% calcium.

Make sure that labeling offers full disclosure of all ingredients including excipients.[hh] They should also have accurate batch numbers and expiration dates and their full address on the bottle. Don't select supplements from companies that only have a P.O. Box address, or worse, no address at all.

If you don't want to do the research necessary to organize your own wellness program, find a wellness consultant, physician or comparably trained person to help you.[ii]

> ***"Choose what is best; habit will soon render it agreeable and easy."***—*Pythagorus (2,500 years ago)*

[hh] Excipients are the fillers added to help make the tablet absorable.
[ii] I am still accepting new clients for consultation, in person, by phone or e-mail. See About Author in the back of this book.

MINERALS

Minerals will be listed by the highest amount found in the body. Not including phosphorus, chloride and sodium which are usually too high in our diet and should not be added.

Calcium—See Calcium chapter: Why Supplements? Diseases related to calcium **deficiency**:

1. Osteoporosis
2. Arthritis
3. Tooth loss
4. Kidney stones
5. Bone spurs
6. High blood pressure
7. Cancer
8. Heart disease

The Standard American Diet ☹ raises our need for calcium. High animal protein diets, high fat diets, high sodium and soda pop take calcium from our bones and teeth.

Potassium—deficiency causes muscle cramps and weakness and heart problems. Good sources are potato skins, fruits and vegetables, legumes, nuts and seeds. According to Julian Whitaker, M.D., consuming more sodium than potassium is a major contributor to cancer, heart disease and high blood pressure. Researchers recommend consuming 5 to 50 times as much potassium as sodium. Most fruits and vegetables have more than 50 times the potassium as sodium.

Magnesium is so important and ignored, it has its own chapter.

Sulfur—deficiency can cause connective tissue problems. Connective tissue helps hold our tissues together so they don't sag. Good sources are protein, garlic, onions and cruciferous vegetables.

Silicon—essential for connective tissues including hair, skin and nails. High in whole grains (the bran part of the grain), only 2% remaining in milled grains.

Microminerals (measured in milligrams[ij])

Iron—essential for preventing anemia. We don't need meat to get iron. **Almonds have 25% more iron than lean beef.** Kelp has 10 times as much iron as liver. Blackstrap molasses has more than 4 times the iron of beef and 10 times the iron of chicken.

Fluoride—strengthens bone and teeth. Found in black tea, some natural water sources and foods grown in high fluoride water and soil.

Zinc—90% of older Americans don't get the RDA for zinc. It is needed for a multitude of bodily functions including immunity, healing, sexual problems and just about everything associated with aging. Deficiency can cause loss of smell and taste, it can also prevent the body from fighting bacterial and viral infections. It is hard to get enough zinc in a good diet. Eating two brazil nuts daily helps add zinc. Brewer's yeast is a good source. Supplementing with 15-30 mg depending on diet should be plenty. For supplements, zinc oxide or sulfate are poorly absorbed. The best supplements are zinc bonded to an amino acid or other natural molecule.

---

[j] A nickel weigh 5 grams, there are 1000 milligrams(mg) in a gram, 1000 micrograms(mcg) in a milligram.

Strontium—important for bones and teeth. Not much is known about this micromineral.

Copper—works in balance with zinc. Too much zinc will cause a deficiency in copper. Nut milk[kk] is high in copper and zinc, two cups a day should prevent deficiency of both. Dark green leafy vegetables and black pepper are good sources. Dr. Joel Wallach author of *Rare Earths,* has stated that gray hair and ptosis are caused by copper deficiency. Ptosis is sagging tissue—eye lids, skin, breasts, stomach etc.

Trace Minerals (measured in micrograms)

Cobalt—Essential part of vitamin B_{12} carnivores (meat eaters) get plenty. Vegetarians can get it from algaes.

Vanadium—helps control blood sugar and decreases cholesterol. High in olive oil and buckwheat.

Iodine—essential for thyroid function and thus all the body's metabolism. Kelp is an excellent source of iodine, calcium, potassium and has 20 times as much iron as beef.

Tin—deficiency causes male baldness and hearing loss. Since it is relatively toxic rely on what you get in plant sources.

Selenium—a powerful antioxidant and rejuvenator. Jean Carper in her book *Stop Aging Now* states "If you don't get enough selenium, your cells fall prey to viruses, cancer, heart disease and signs of rapid aging. To keep your youth, take a low-level selenium supplement, as many research scientists do." Selenium content of food is strongly dependent on soil content. Brazil nuts that come in

---

[kk] See the Recipe chapter.

the shell (grown in Brazilian forests) generally have more than a days supply in 2 nuts (200mcg.). Shelled nuts are grown in lower selenium soils and have about 25mcg. per nut. Other good sources are garlic and organically grown tomatoes.

Manganese—important in a variety of the body's enzyme systems including hormone synthesis, energy production and neurotransmitter formation. It may prevent Parkinson's disease. High in nuts, bran from several grains, spinach, tea, cocoa and beets.

Nickel—deficiency causes poor growth. Found in legumes, whole grains and walnuts.

Molybdenum—helps prevent cancer and premature death. Found in a whole plant food diet if soils are not depleted.

Chromium—is essential for blood sugar control, it also helps to maintain muscle and lose fat. Chromium deficiency is common because of depleted soils and not eating enough whole plant foods. Scientists at the USDA designed a super diet to increase chromium intake. With their best effort a 2,000 calorie diet only contained 48 mg., 1/4 of what is needed for optimal health.

Laboratory rats normally live 2 1/2 years; when fed modest amounts of chromium they lived 1 year longer. In humans, this would mean living past 100 years. Chromium keeps our insulin efficient and controls blood sugar. Part of the aging process is caused by glycosylation of body proteins (sugar crosslinking). Chromium also increases artery cleaning HDL by 11- 20% it decreases total cholesterol by over 14%.

Chromium increases the master hormone DHEA by about 10%. DHEA is a marker of human aging, it declines as we age, at age 70 we have 10% of what we had at 25. DHEA is becoming a popular anti-aging supplement prescribed by doctors.[ll]

Chromate or solgar GTF chromium are probably the best sources, picolinate has recently been associated with tumors in rats (at extremely high doses). 200-400mcg. is needed daily.

Boron—helps to prevent osteoporosis, arthritis and high blood pressure. Good sources are apples, grapes, broccoli and whole foods.

Other important minerals

Silver—kills over 650 disease causing organisms.

Germanium—high in garlic and ginseng. Enhances immune system function.

Lithium, Gallium, Bismuth, Cesium, Europium, Gold, Lanthanum, Neodymium, Praseodymium, Antimony, Samarium, Thulium, Yttrium—most of these doubled the life span of laboratory animals as well as help prevent cancer and other diseases. Don't expect to find these in commercially grown foods. I take essential colloidal minerals and high mineral content algae to get these and all the other minerals in my diet.[mm]

The best recipe for getting these minerals is my nutmilk recipe found in the recipe chapter. Mineral content of the 3 main ingredients:

[ll] See the chapter: Reversing The Aging Process
[mm] See the resource directory in the back of this book.

Minerals	Almonds 1/2 cup	Flax[nn] 2 rounded Tbls.	Tofu 1 cup
Calcium	210mg.	40mg.	272mg.
Phosphorus	360mg.	120mg.	200mg.
Potassium	550mg.	140mg.	high
Sulfur	?	55mg.	?
Magnesium	200	100mg.	150mg.
Iron	2.5mg.	1.8mg.	9mg.
Fluoride	65mcg.	?	?
Zinc	3mg.	10mg.	3.5mg.
Manganese	1.5mg.	high	high
Copper	0.8mg.	1mg.	1mg..
Protein[oo]	12gm.	7gm.	25gm.
Fiber	5gm.	8.1gm.	none

Fluoride, selenium, molybdenum and chromium content are dependent on the soil and water they were grown in. Nickel is supplied by the walnuts.

[nn] Omega Fortified Flax
[oo] The protein in these 3 combined are complete and easier for the body to digest and absorb than meat.

MAGNESIUM— THE MIRACLE MINERAL

Magnesium is the single most important mineral to add to your diet, even more so than calcium or zinc. Julian Whitaker, M.D. states that if he were limited to one mineral supplement it would be magnesium.

Magnesium is essential to prevent premature aging, animals fed diets deficient in magnesium aged rapidly and died younger. **Magnesium deficiency has been linked to several diseases:**

Problems That May Be Helped With Magnesium

High Blood Pressure	Heart Disease
Kidney Stones	Hyperactivity
Autism	PMS
Epilepsy	Menstrual Pain
Muscle Cramps	Insomnia
Osteoporosis	Anxiety
Depression	Fatigue
Alcoholism	Aging
Diabetes	Vascular Spasms
Cancer	Stress
Headaches	Muscle Weakness

Most Americans are deficient in magnesium—According to Jean Carper, author of *Stop Aging Now*, and numerous other authorities, 75% of adult Americans are falling short of the Recommended Dietary Allowance for magnesium. Elson M. Haas, M.D. also states that many authorities recommend twice the RDA. By these standards, anyone whose diet lacks high magnesium food, should take magnesium supplements.

Causes of deficiency—The Standard American Diet (SAD) is sadly lacking in magnesium. This deficiency is not only from lack of consuming high magnesium foods but also due to food processing. Sherry Rogers, M.D., reported in the International Medicine World Report in 1992 that 75% of magnesium is lost with food processing. 80% of magnesium is lost by removing the germ and bran of whole grains. White or the so-called enriched wheat flour,[PP] robs your body of magnesium. Carbohydrate metabolism depends on magnesium as does most energy requiring reactions in the body. Muscle contraction depends on magnesium, especially the heart muscle.

Other causes of deficiency include eating foods from magnesium poor soils. Drinking soft water. Consumption of alcohol, caffeine and sugar. One 12 oz. Soda pop can bind 30 mg. of magnesium and flush it out of the body. Fatty food decreases the absorption of magnesium to as little as 1% being utilized by the body. Exercise can lead to magnesium loss. Athletes and others can suffer a loss of magnesium through sweat. This loss can bring fatigue and muscle cramps.

Drugs which can deplete magnesium levels include: birth control pills, amphotericin B, cyclosporine, cisplatin, gentamicin, diuretics, pentamidine and others.

Testing for deficiency—according to Dr. Robert M. McLean of the Yale School of Medicine. Dr. McLean also stated that the amount of magnesium in the blood does not necessarily correlate with the amount of the mineral stored in the body, "making a magnesium deficiency difficult to pinpoint."

Aging—magnesium deficiency induces rapid aging by allowing more free radical damage inside our cells. (See the chapter on reversing the aging process). According to French researchers,

---

[PP] Essentially white flour with 12 vitamins added.

magnesium deficiency allows "uncontrolled calcium inflow" which is a "central event in the aging process and cell injury."

The powerhouses of our cells are the mitochondria. They provide the energy to run almost all the body's functions. Mitochondria require an abundance of magnesium to function properly, without adequate amounts damage occurs. Free radical experts believe the number one cause of aging is damage to the mitochondria.

High Blood Pressure—is often treated with dangerous drugs called calcium channel blockers. These toxic chemicals alter the access of calcium into cells. This relaxes the smooth muscle of arterial walls which in turn reduces blood pressure. Magnesium does the same thing without the dangerous side effects.

Heart Disease—Epidemiological studies have shown that populations that consume higher amounts of magnesium have less heart disease and high blood pressure problems. Over half of the patients in one cardiac unit had low magnesium levels in their blood. Magnesium protects the heart in several ways. Magnesium can prevent vascular spasms, correct arrythmias and prevent abnormal blood clotting. Magnesium increases the survival from heart attacks. In one study, magnesium was given to 50 patients and only one died. The other group of 53 was given a placebo and nine died. In several studies magnesium performed better at controlling cardiac arrhythmias than the usual drugs.

High Cholesterol—rabbits on a normal cholesterol diet were given five times the RDA of magnesium. This resulted in a 30-40 % drop in their blood cholesterol and other blood fats as compared to a low magnesium diet.

Diabetes—90% of diabetic patients are magnesium deficient because of the disease and the drugs used to treat it. Both insulin and diuretics deplete the body's magnesium. Diabetic patients with the lowest magnesium are at the greatest risk for retinal bleeding and all the complications of deficiency listed above. Robert K. Rude, M.D. favors a 300 to 400 mg. supplement of magnesium to correct diabetic deficiencies. He also states that diabetes is characterized by magnesium depletion.

Asthma—Because of magnesium's ability to relax smooth muscle, it is quite effective at opening the contracted bronchioles of an asthmatic.

Leg Cramps—Dr. Richard Rivlin at Memorial Sloan-Kettering Cancer Center (NY) says "the prevalence of heart disease, diabetes and even leg cramps increases dramatically among older persons, and these are all health conditions in which magnesium deficiency has been found."

Chronic Fatigue Syndrome—The CFS Research Foundation reported in their publication "Health Watch", that a combination of magnesium and malic acid (extracted from apples and other foods) has been useful in treating some people with CFS. Dr. Daniel Peterson says that up to 40% of CFS patients find benefit from this treatment; but that patients may take two weeks to respond to this treatment. The therapeutic dose recommended is 6-12 tablets/day of malic acid and magnesium hydroxide.

The magazine "Better Nutrition for Today's Living" also reported that CFS patients should consider supplementing their diet with vitamin B12, high doses of vitamins C, E, beta carotene and CoQ10.

Energy/Fatigue—At least 50% of adults seeking medical treatment complain of fatigue. In many cases, fatigue can be relieved by a combination of magnesium aspartate and potassium aspartate; increasing capacity for prolonged exercise up to 50%.

PMS—According to Elson M. Haas, M.D., "Menstrual cramps, irritability, fatigue, depression and water retention have been lessened with magnesium along with calcium and often with vitamin B$_6$"

Kidney Stones—research has shown that adequate magnesium intake helps to block the formation of kidney stones.

Children—have been treated for both autism and hyperactivity with magnesium and vitamin B$_6$ according to Dr. Haas.

Magnesium sources—Food sources high in magnesium include dark green, leafy vegetables, nuts, flaxseed, whole grains, legumes, apples, bananas and grapefruit; sources with moderate magnesium include fruits, vegetables, meats and fish and those low in magnesium include dairy products. Five figs provide 20% of the RDA of magnesium, calcium and iron.

Supplement sources include magnesium salts of chloride, gluconate, lactate, aspartate, hydroxide and oxide salts. Oxide and hydroxide salts are the least absorbed.

Different magnesium salts have different biological effects. Magnesium aspartate has demonstrated beneficial effects beyond its role as a magnesium source, including superior protection from antioxidant damage, "anti-fatigue" effects, cholesterol lowering effects, activation of cellular respiration and excellent absorption, particularly when combined with potassium aspartate.

All it takes to get the RDA of magnesium is to eat one of these or a combination:
- 4 oz. of almonds
- 4 oz of molasses
- 5 oz wheat germ
- 6 oz of soybeans
- 12 oz whole grains

This is why I strongly recommend replacing dairy products with my nut milk recipe.[99]

Dosage:
National Research Council recommends:

Children Age 0-10	150-250 mg.
Adults	300-400 mg.
Pregnant/Lactating Women	450 mg.

Dr. Mildred Seelig, as reported in the Journal of the American College of Nutrition (Vol.13, No.5, 429-446 (1994), feels that an intake of 6-10 mg. per kilogram of weight is optimal and feels that the RDA listed above is too low (5 mg./kg/day).

"Extensive data suggests that if the calcium/magnesium ratio exceeds 2:1, cardiovascular death is positively correlated with rising calcium/magnesium ratio." Dr. Seelig quotes an article in *Advances in Cardiology* (1978) by Karpannen stating that there is a direct correlation of rising IHD (ischemic heart disease) with increasing calcium/ magnesium ratios. Finland, with a 4:1 ratio has the highest rate of "sudden coronary death", USA is next with a 3:1 ratio; Japan, Greece and Yugoslavia have the lowest IHD rate and lowest calcium/magnesium ratio. "It appears that the National Institute of Health's recommendation of calcium intake of 1500 mg./day may increase substantially the cardiac death rate in this country because it destroys the proper Ca/ mg. ratio."

If a person takes 1,200 mg./day of calcium and gets the normal magnesium dose of 300 mg./day through diet, the ratio is 4:1; if the calcium goes to 1,500 mg. and the magnesium stays at 300 mg. the ratio becomes 5:1. It seems obvious that caution should be taken when increasing calcium without magnesium.

A study done by Dr. R. B. Singh in India in which he gave one group 1,142 mg./day of magnesium for ten years and a control

---

[99] See chapter: Recipes

group received 418 mg./day of magnesium. This study showed the higher intake group had a much lower death rate.

Toxicity—in the presence of normal renal function, excess dietary magnesium virtually never occurs. Diarrhea is the most common side effect and it stops with a decrease in magnesium use.

Absorption—The July, 1993 issue of *Nutritional News* states that "magnesium absorption from the gastrointestinal tract is essentially limited to the small intestine. In the normal individual, approximately fifty percent of ingested magnesium is absorbed. The intake of magnesium, however, alters absorption. On a high magnesium diet, as little as twenty-five percent may be absorbed, while up to seventy-five percent of ingested magnesium may be absorbed on a low magnesium diet."

If you take 1,000 mg./day of magnesium you may only absorb 25% or 250 mg. of the 1,000 mg., yet if you take 250 mg./day of magnesium you may absorb as much as 187.50 mg. of the 250 mg.

In addition, the article also says "the absorption of magnesium decreases rapidly when doses are greater than 200 mg." (increasing risk of loose stools and diarrhea).

Summary:
1. Follow the rejuvenation diet,[π] you will have no problems with magnesium deficiency, especially if you use nutmilk recipe.
2. When you are not following the diet take potassium and magnesium aspartate between meals.
3. If you take calcium, make sure you get at least half as much magnesium, more if you use dairy products or think you may be currently magnesium deficient.
4. Divide your daily dose into segments of 200mg or less to reduce chance of loose stools/diarrhea.
5. Persons with impaired renal function or kidney disease **must** check with their physician before adding magnesium supplements.

[π] See the chapter : Diet.

THE B VITAMINS

In the summer of 1979 in the U.C. Davis library I felt inspired to pickup a magazine to read. The magazine was *Atlantic Monthly,* May, 1979. This was the first time I saw the *Atlantic Monthly.* I read the most amazing article. It described how a simple vitamin deficiency caused arteriosclerosis. The vitamin was vitamin B_6, is a necessary cofactor in the conversion of homocysteine (HC) to cystathionine. Folic acid, riboflavin (vitamin B_2) and cobalamin (B_{12}) likewise participate in the re-methylation of most HC back into methionine, which is not dangerous when B_6 is adequate. Homocysteine results from normal metabolism of methionine, abundant in red meat and milk products. Research has shown even slightly elevated HC is an independent risk factor for heart disease and stroke. If elevated, it puts one at risk without respect to age, diabetes, smoking or any other conventional risk factor.

Although HC's concentration is only about one thousandth that of cholesterol, it promotes the tiny clots that initiate arterial damage, as well as catastrophic clotting that precipitates most heart attacks and strokes, arterial spasms, aneurysms, obesity, cancer and much more. HC does its deadly work by oxidizing cholesterol.[π]

Cholesterol is not the villain it has been portrayed to be except for less than 1% of the population that has a family tendency to ultra-high cholesterol levels. Cholesterol doesn't damage arteries until it is oxidized. Cholesterol molecules combine with oxygen molecules forming oxysterols, or oxyradicals. These are carried by the low density lipoproteins (LDLs), which are then only accomplices in arterial damage through oxidative modification of arterial walls. Damage is proportional to oxysterols' concentration

---

[π] Joseph G. Hattersley, *Vitamin B_6: The Overlooked Key To Preventing Heart Attacks.*

and at autopsy atherosclerosis correlates with the accumulation of lipid peroxides and hydroperoxides in serum and atheromas.

Other producers of oxysterols are polyunsaturated oils, partially hydrogenated oils, free radicals and oxidized food.[ss] Pre-formed oxysterols are in processed foods (foods that have been exposed to high heat and oxygen). Some examples are powdered milk or egg, partially hydrogenated oils (found in the majority of packaged supermarket foods). These deadly fats are found in high amounts in "fast foods". The French fries at McDonalds, Burger King and most chain restaurants are worse for your arteries than the hamburgers. Oxysterols like cholesterol serve important functions in the body, it is not until they reach high levels that they become damaging. After eating processed foods they may reach levels 1,000 times normal.

The good news is vitamin B_6 seems to be the "magic bullet." In studies that include the only change as adding vitamin B_6, participants have had less cardiovascular disease. Vitamin B_6's action are not all known, it acts as an antioxidant, a antihistamine and is a co-factor in the metabolism and biochemistry of most food components including most amino acids, fatty acids and sugars.

Joseph G. Hattersley wrote an article about vitamin B_6, *Vitamin B_6: The Overlooked Key To Preventing Heart Attacks*, he cited over 80 research articles. In the article he says, "Expanded food fortification should include folate, vitamin B_{12} (cobalamin) and at least magnesium and zinc. Vitamin C intakes should be raised to tenfold the RDA and an equivalent amount of bioflavonoids (which may double the efficacy of ascorbic acid) should be added. These nutrients, ingested from inception, might end the 20th century's epidemic of heart attacks, strokes and cardiac arrests in about two generations. Because all degenerative diseases "have on the membrane level and on the genetic level, very

---

[ss] See the chapters Reversing the Aging Process, Deadly Fats vs. Healing Fats.

much a common denominator", this program should also lower the incidence of such diseases as diabetes and cancer."

Depending on your diet, health and biochemical individuality 5-50 mg of vitamin B_6 two to three times a day should be all that is necessary to maintain optimal health. Vitamin B_6 also needs folate, magnesium and vitamins B-2 and B_{12} to function optimally (without these accessory nutrients neurological side effects may occur at doses over 200 mg daily). I recommend 400 to 800 mcgs of folate, a vitamin B complex with a minimum of 5 mg of all the B vitamins (thiamin B_1, riboflavin B_2, niacin B_3 and pantothenic acid B_5) 2 to 3 times a day and vitamin B_{12} is best taken sublingually 500 mcgs once a week or daily if needed. Other B vitamins include choline and biotin.[tt]

As powerful as B_6 is let's not forget a mostly vegetarian diet, exercise and other important supplements.

Alan Gaby, M.D. in his book, *B_6: The Natural Healer,* (Keats Publishing). Dr. Gaby believes we have increased needs for B_6 based on increased health problems related to B_6. Some health problems, such as carpal tunnel syndrome, were rarely reported 60 years ago. Other examples include kidney stones (doubled in the past 30 years), hyperactivity (also known as attention deficit disorder, affects 5-20% of all children, not a major problem 20 years ago) and PMS (affects up to 90% of all American women). B_6 is also involved (either as a reducer of risk factors or as therapy) in heart disease, elevated cholesterol, platelet adhesiveness (stroke risk factor), bladder cancer, glucose tolerance problems (blood sugar), lupus (SLE), B_6-responsive arthritis, alcoholism, dental cavities, MSG sensitivity and asthma.

What has happened in the past half century that might explain why we are seeing a rash of health problems that respond to

---

[tt] You get both of these in sufficient quantities in my nutmilk recipe.

vitamin B_6 therapy? First, we are processing the food more and throwing away the parts that are rich in B_6. While processed food and increased amounts of sugar in the diet, account for part of the problem, they are not enough to explain why people seem to need so much more B_6 today. The second part of the problem may be the key. There are chemicals in our food that use up our bodies stores of B_6. When a chemical interferes with a nutrient the body needs, it's called an antimetabolite. Antimetabolites of B_6 can cause problems in several ways: They might interfere with the absorption of B_6, cause it to be used up more quickly, or damage it so it won't work correctly. In other words, the antimetabolites work against the normal action of B_6. When this happens, our bodies need more B_6. What are some of these antimetabolites of B_6? The known list is small. As time goes on, we will probably find more and more things that not only interfere with vitamin B_6, but also increase our need for other vitamins and minerals. Two known antimetabolites are hydrazine or hydrazide. These compounds look a little like B_6. Sometimes, Dr. Gaby points out, when one chemical looks like another chemical, the body can't easily distinguish between them. When the body can't tell the difference, it might try to substitute the false compound for the nutrient. When this happens, the antimetabolite can interfere with the body's use of the real vitamin. Hydrazines and hydrazides are common in the environment. They appear in herbicides (sprayed on tobacco, potatoes and onions), field sprays (to help ripen peaches, nectarines, tomatoes, Brussels sprouts, cherries, grapes and apples), rocket and jet exhaust (traces can hang around for days or weeks after the jet flies by), cigarette smoke, some prescription medications (for tuberculosis, depression, heart problems and high blood pressure) and food coloring (yellow number 5).

Scientists know that other things besides hydrazines and hydrazides, can increase our need for B_6. For example, birth control pills, PCB's (polychlorinated biphenyls used in transformers and capacitors which are contaminating our water and food), heated vegetable oil and other by-products of food processing. The list goes on, everywhere we turn we seem to run into something that interferes with our body's normal healthy use of B_6. As a physician, this suggests that even if you don't have a specific problem you can relate to B_6 deficiency, you would be smart to take a supplement that contains B_6. In fact, the evidence is building that so many chemicals are now in our environment that have never been part of human ecology before, and that many of them interfere with or create a higher requirement for vitamins and minerals. It may be that nutritional supplements are less a luxury and more a necessity for good health now than ever before.[uu]

Premenstrual syndrome (PMS) is a common complaint for women. The usual prescribed medicines don't get to the underlying problem and often don't even help the symptoms. Women who turn to alternative treatment get mixed results. In studies in England, it was found that a vast majority of women with PMS who took up to 400-600 mg of B_6 daily had all their symptoms relieved. Follow-up studies showed none of the women had any side effects.

Carpal tunnel syndrome, CTS (where some fingers in the hand get numb and tingly because of pressure on the median nerve) is practically always relieved by B_6. The dosage level for CTS is between 300 to 600 mg. According to Drs. Wright and Gaby, this dose needs to be maintained for 10-12 weeks in order for tissue to become sufficiently saturated.

Michael Lesser, M. D., in his book *Nutrition and Vitamin Therapy*, reports that 10 mg. of vitamin B_6 and 300 mg. of magnesium oxide prevented recurrence of kidney and urinary tract stones in 80% of patients with a long history of the disease. Dr.

[uu] See the chapter: Why Supplements?

Lesser also reports that this combination was helpful in treating hyperactive children.

Vitamin B_6 more than any other B vitamin supports the immune system fight infections and cancer.

NATURE'S REJUVENATOR
GINKGO BILOBA

Slow Down the Aging Process with Nature's Natural Remedy

The ginkgo is the world's oldest living species of tree, traced back more than 200 million years (the Permian Period). This tree was almost lost to humkankind during the Ice Age, but fortunately survived in some areas of China. The ginkgo tree has shown a remarkable resilience and resistance to insects, disease, and pollution. For this reason, ginkgo trees are now frequently planted along major boulevards and streets in cities throughout the world.

I believe that ginkgo biloba is one of the best herbs to prevent and reverse the aging process. At a cellular level, ginkgo generally protects against structural attack by free radicals, stabilizes membranes and helps to "tune-up energy production" in the mitochondria of the cell. Ginkgo has been proven effective both against peripheral vascular disorders and against disorders of the cerebral circulation. It protects capillaries against becoming fragile or leaking blood into the tissues. Ginkgo also protects circulating blood against pooling and the formation of clots.

Ginkgo's greatest benefits are improving circulation to the places we need it the most brain, nervous system, heart, eyes, inner ear, penis, feet and hands.

Ginkgo appears to have a three-pronged benefit:
1. **Dilation of constricted blood vessels,** resulting in greater delivery of blood to the tissues and better drainage of wastes, particularly through arteries partially blocked by atherosclerosis.

2. **Inhibition of platelet aggregation,** discouraging circulating platelets from clumping at points of "wear and tear" on the walls of aging blood vessels.
3. **Protection from aging by protecting the body from oxidation.**

The Ginkgo biloba tree is the oldest surviving species of tree on earth. Ginkgo has flourished almost unchanged since 150 million years ago (during the Mesozoic period, when dinosaurs roamed the Earth), and its ancestors can be traced back 250 million years. Ginkgo survived changing climatic and geologic conditions, including ice ages and at least two catastrophic extinction's of a major percentage of then thriving species. Ginkgo survived only in China, where it was later cultivated as a sacred tree.

Ginkgo is a living lesson in vitality to those observing its nature: it is extremely long-lived with trees surviving as long as 1,000 years, growing to a height of 100-122 feet with a diameter of 3-4 feet. The ginkgo tree is significantly resistant to infection, resilient against both parasites and pollution in the cities where it lines the boulevards. In fact, ginkgo trees are so hardy that a solitary ginkgo was the only tree to survive the atomic blast in Hiroshima. You can still see this tree alive today, standing near the epicenter of the blast site, a living testament to the ginkgo's remarkable ability to survive.

It was the Chinese who first discovered the healing properties of this beneficial tree. The ancient Chinese made preparations of dried ginkgo leaves to treat symptoms of aging such as poor circulation, memory loss, and general mental deterioration. They also used ginkgo nuts for thousands of years as a remedy for cancer, venereal disease, asthma, lung weakness and congestion, impaired hearing and to increase sexual energy and generally promote longevity.

Today, ginkgo biloba is one of Europe's most widely prescribed botanicals, 10 million prescriptions per year with sales reaching about $500 million annually.

Dr. Schwabe developed the standardized concentrated extract of ginkgo biloba leaves (24 percent flavone glycosides) known in Europe as EGB761, marketed under the names Tebonin and Rokan (Germany), and Tanakan (France).

There are many other ginkgo extracts coming from Europe and Asia that are still standardized to the 24% content of flavone glycosides established by the original Schwabe product. Their ratios of flavonoid, ginkgolide and bilobalide content can sometimes vary. Achieving the ideal balance of these important constituents was thought by Schwabe to be essential in assuring the effectiveness of the final extract.

The ginkgo biloba extract only remains in the body for a short time, it is rapidly absorbed and has a half life of approximately 3 hours. That's one reason why most of the scientific studies involved three daily dosages of the ginkgo biloba extract (GBE). The 27-step extraction process requires 50 pounds of dried leaves to yield 1 pound of the standardized extract and takes up to two weeks to complete.

The compounds most responsible for ginkgo's effectiveness are the flavone glycosides (sugars derived from the chemical of the natural color of the leaf—flavo is a prefix indicating yellow; ginkgo leaves turn yellow-gold in the fall), including kaempferol, quercetin, isorhamnetin, and also proanthocyanidins. These compounds contribute to ginkgo biloba's powerful antioxidant and free radical scavenging properties.

Recent research focuses on a set of alcohol-soluble terpenes, the most important of which are known as ginkgolides and bilobalides. These compounds, unique to ginkgo, show positive benefits in improving circulation, decreasing blood viscosity and decreasing tissue damage during inflammation.

During the last fifty years, the hundreds of scientific studies on the ginkgo biloba extract have been conducted in Germany and France (and a few in Italy, Japan and China), and the physiological effects of ginkgo have been shown to be many and varied.

Mental Health

Biologically, the human aging process begins accelerating after age 30. Part of this process appears to involve a gradual loss of brain cells. It has been estimated that 50,000 neurons (brain cells) deteriorate daily, beginning at age 20. So by the time we are 70 years old, we could lose almost 10 percent of our original brain cell count. The flow of blood through the brain also slows down through the years as a result of deposits on the walls of the blood vessels. The combination of these two factors can contribute to a number of problems, including diminished memory function—it can be very frustrating to feel like your memory may be slipping. European studies show that ginkgo increases blood flow in the brain, helps prevent and treat stroke and improves memory and mental prowess.

Cerebral Insufficiency—is a term for a condition that includes a general lack of mental health and vitality, particularly in people over 70.

Ginkgo's spectacular rise in popularity over the last 15 years has been due, in part, to its documented ability to increase circulation to the brain and to the extremities. Studies have indicated that by age 70, blood flow to the brain is reduced by 20 percent. Individuals showing signs of dementia (including Alzheimer's disease) may have a reduction of over 30 percent. Proper circulation to the brain ensures sufficient delivery not only of oxygen, but also of glucose, the brain's primary fuel. It follows that optimal brain function depends on a large and constant supply of glucose and oxygen. Without these important circulation dependent substances, a long list of conditions, including memory loss, decrease
in alertness and concentration, dizziness, vertigo, depression, headache and tinnitus, can result.

In a study conducted by Dr. Weitbrecht and Dr. Jansen of Germany. The study consisted of 40 patients, aged 60-80 years, who had been diagnosed with various levels of dementia. The patients were split into two groups, with one group receiving a daily dose of ginkgo biloba extract and the other group receiving a placebo. The two groups were monitored for three months.

At the end of the trial, those patients given the ginkgo extract showed a significant improvement both on mental skill tests and on their emotional outlook. All exhibited a marked improvement in their mental capacity, mental alertness, sociability and mood. Those given the placebos, however, showed no such improvements.

Another similar study by a medical researcher, Dr. G. Vorberg, involved 112 patients ranging in ages from 55 to 94. These patients all exhibited various degrees of mental deterioration and were diagnosed with chronic cerebral insufficiency. Each patient was administered ginkgo biloba daily for one year and then reevaluated. The results showed a significant improvement in mental performance and vigilance in the patients, along with increased cognitive function.

In a year-long study directed by Sitzer (1987), ginkgo extract proved, once again, to be effective in treating cerebral insufficiency. A group of 30 patients with symptoms such as headache, vertigo and tinnitus were given a 40 mg dose of ginkgo extract 3 times a day. The researchers found a "very strong improvement" in these symptoms after only 2 to 4 months of treatment, and the patients "kept on improving during the course of the year."

For cerebral impairment due to degenerative or vascular causes, the average success rate in several open, non-comparative studies was found to be 60 to 78 percent. In these studies, which had no control group, the ginkgo extract was administered orally over periods of 3 weeks to 1 year, at doses of 120 to 360 mg per day.

More carefully controlled, double-blind studies for the same condition confirmed these findings. In a total of 9 studies, which lasted from 5 weeks to 12 months, the overall improvement rate for patients who took ginkgo extract was between 44 and 92 percent, while people who took placebos showed only a 14 to 44 percent rate of improvement—quite a significant difference.

Another study, conducted by Dr. D. M. Warburton, of the University of Reading, England, examined 20 clinical applications of ginkgo used by patients with vascular brain disorders, dementia and cognitive dysfunction. In all cases the ginkgo users showed a marked improvement in mental alertness, short-term memory, communication, freedom from confusion and a wide variety of other recuperative effects. In particular, those patients who originally exhibited the worst symptoms ultimately showed the most significant improvements.

Short-term Memory Improvement

Several clinical studies have shown that ginkgo extracts improve short-term memory.

One double-blind study was performed with six human volunteers, it was found that a single 600 mg dose of ginkgo enhanced the speed of information recall from short-term memory. Doses of 120 or 240 mg of ginkgo extract as well as doses of placebo did not lead to an improvement in short term memory. This study as well as several other related clinical studies show the efficacy of ginkgo biloba extract on improving neural function and nervous system tone.

A second study (also double-blind), eight healthy female volunteers took various doses of ginkgo extracts or placebo. After giving the volunteers a battery of memory tests, the researchers found that short-term memory was "very significantly improved" only in the subjects who took ginkgo. The authors of this German study concluded by saying, "These results differentiate ginkgo biloba extract from sedative and stimulant drugs and suggest a specific effect on memory processes." Thus ginkgo seems to enhance memory by acting directly on the "central cognitive processes" in the brain.

Due to ginkgo's ability to increase blood flow to the brain and therefore improve delivery of oxygen and glucose, the standardized extract has become one of the **leading medicines in the world for treatment of diminished mental function in elderly patients.** Patients with early signs of impaired memory and mental performance have shown dramatic clinical improvement once started on the ginkgo extract. Evidence also suggests that **taking the extract prior to these changes associated with aging may actually delay or inhibit their onset.**

Peripheral Arterial Insufficiency
In my practice, I see many patients with nerve and vascular problems. These problems are usually related to diabetes, smoking or eating the SAD diet. Their primary care physicians have usually prescribed drugs including anti-depressants, often the patient received no relief. I always recommend ginkgo along with other herbs, vitamins, minerals and foods. It is better to treat the cause rather than the symptoms. Most of my patients have improved when standard drug therapy failed.

When cholesterol deposits narrow the arteries in the legs, the result is intermittent claudication (lameness), limping, pain, cramping and weakness, particularly in the thighs and calves of the elderly.

An example of ginkgo's ability to relieve vascular problems in limbs can be seen in a clinical trial conducted at the Maria-Hilf Hospital in Germany. In this six-month study, patients suffering from claudication and other vascular problems were administered ginkgo biloba extract daily.

At the end of the trial, those patients suffering from grade II lower limb arteritis (inflammation of an artery) showed over a 100 percent improvement in their condition. The patients were able to walk with complete freedom from pain.

Those patients suffering from Raynaud's disease (intermittent attacks of a decreased blood supply to extremities such as fingers, toes, ears and nose) showed a 33 percent improvement.

Another German study conducted two years later involving patients suffering from claudication had similar results, with some patients reporting a resolution to other minor circulatory ailments, as well.

In one impressive study, with 79 patients diagnosed with arteriopathy (a diseased state of the arteries) in the lower limbs, half of the group was given ginkgo extract (40 mg dose 3x/day), while the other half was given a placebo. Using both objective and subjective measures of improvement, a highly significant increase in the ability to walk for distance without pain was found in the ginkgo group only. In this study and others, ginkgo extract also reduced cramping and numbness of the extremities.

The clinical demonstration that ginkgo biloba extract improved limb blood flow, together with improved walking tolerance indicated that the extract may be the botanical supplement of choice in peripheral arterial insufficiency.

The Heart & Vascular Integrity

Ginkgo improves blood flow to the heart and appears to reduce heart attack risk by preventing the formation of blood clots in the coronary arteries. A study conducted in Germany documented the benefits of long-term use of ginkgo in reducing cardiovascular risk, including those associated with coronary heart disease, hypertension, hypercholesterolemia and diabetes mellitus.

Clinical research also renders evidence that ginkgo protects vascular integrity including protection against leakiness of tiny vessels and spasms of the arteries. Ginkgo widens blood vessels and tiny capillaries and increases the flexibility or "muscle tone" of blood vessels—even the blood cells, themselves.

Spasms in the small arteries in the brain reduce the blood flow to the brain and can be quite harmful. These spasms can be caused by a variety of factors and conditions, but may be mediated by neurotransmitters, the chemical "messengers" that relay nerve impulses from one nerve cell to another. If such spasms occur during conditions of reduced oxygen supply, the negative effects may be compounded.

Ginkgo extract has demonstrated a relaxing effect on the arteries and arterioles (smaller branches than arteries) which may even be strong enough to counteract vascular spasms. By doing so, ginkgo also improves blood circulation. For instance, in another study in which ginkgo extract was given intravenously to 12 patients with cerebrovascular disease, it was found that "cerebral perfusion" (blood flow through brain tissue) was increased by over 8 percent—not only in healthy tissue, but in damaged areas as well. This means that ginkgo did not "steal" blood from damaged areas and cause it to be sent to healthy tissue, but actually increased blood flow in the whole area.

"Leakiness" of the tiny capillaries in the brain happens when the walls of the blood vessels start to lose their tone. This condition can result from scarring or damage caused by free radicals or over-activity of the immune system due to stress or a diet high in animal products and hydrogenated "trans-fats". The inflammatory process, which increases secretion of histamine, can be another cause of leakiness. But whatever the cause or combination of causes, leakiness can lead to brain and nerve damage and retinal bleeding. The build up of metabolic wastes can lead to more free radical damage.

Free Radical Scavenger[ww]

Ginkgo acts as a powerful antioxidant or free radical scavenger. Studies in France have shown ginkgo to be very effective in protecting the lipid (fat) portion of cellular membranes from free radical damage. If one considers that the brain and nerve cells contain the highest content of unsaturated fats (lipids) of any cells

---

[ww] See the chapter: Reversing The Aging Process.

in the body, this protective action further supports ginkgo's benefits for the central nervous system.

French researcher K. Drieu notes that "free radicals influence the fluidity and the permeability of [all] cell membranes; these effects have repercussions on capillaries, cells and neurons. A major part of the effect of ginkgo biloba extract seems to be due to a restoration of membrane integrity."

Ginkgo biloba extract has been found to neutralize free radicals and prevent them from damaging the myelin insulation on nerves and other cells in the brain. Ginkgo also prevents free radical damage to the rest of the body's cells and organs.

One of the chemical compounds in ginkgo extracts which are responsible for fighting free-radicals (called flavonoids) were shown in laboratory studies to be up to 10 times more potent free radical scavengers than the flavonoids commonly found in other plant sources, such as citrus peels and many fruits, including blueberries.[xx]

In vitro research has also shown that two substances, which make up 47 percent of the ginkgo extract, the ginkgoheterosides and the proanthocyanidines, are nature's most potent free radical scavengers, one explanation for ginkgo's anti-aging properties.[yy]

Further studies involving diabetic retinopathy also demonstrate the free radical scavenging properties of the ginkgo extract. Experiments using diabetic rats showed the retinas of the group receiving ginkgo extract were in significantly better shape than those of the untreated rats.

Ginkgolides and Platelets
Recently, there has been research on Platelet Activating Factors (PAFs). Just as free radicals, PAFs are formed in the body under poor metabolic conditions, and are at least partially responsible for a number of abnormal physiological situation, such as clotting of

---

[xx] See pg. 186, Bioflavonoids.
[yy] See pg. 189, proanthocyanidins.

the blood (thromboses), bronchoconstriction and shock reaction (both cardiogenic and anaphylactic). PAF is involved in a number of biological processes, such as arterial blood flow, organ graft rejection, asthma attacks, and blood clots involved in heart attacks and some strokes. By inhibiting PAF, ginkgo has great healing potential, particularly in conditions associated with aging.

PAF activates several kinds of immune cells (neutrophils, eosinophils, macrophages) and endothelial cells—all of which secrete chemicals that create inflammation and enhance the blood-clotting process. Chronic stressful conditions, including a diet high in processed oils and exposure to environmental allergens or even food allergens (such as wheat or dairy for some people), can over-stimulate the production of PAF. When PAF in turn activates too many immune cells, the immune system can go haywire, producing conditions such as asthma, toxic shock from bacterial sepsis and maybe even atherosclerosis and stroke. As I mentioned in a previous chapter, free radicals are important to the immune system, free radicals are produced to destroy invading micro-organisms. Unfortunately, if the immune system is too active the fallout, from this "biological warfare" may be challenging for the body to clean up. PAF stimulated cells also produce histamine that increases "leakiness" and prostaglandins that promote inflammation.

PAF plays essential roles in the immune system and is vital in regulating many biochemical processes of the body (such as platelet secretion for initiating the inflammatory response and protection against bacterial invasion), we do not understand all the details of why PAF and other natural "messenger" substances like prostaglandins and histamine go awry and initiate degenerative or disease-promoting activity in the body.

However, we do know that ginkgo extracts hold great promise for protecting against various PAF-induced conditions that arise from over-activation of the immune system. Ginkgo helps control

PAF's influence on the lung, heart, smooth muscles (such as in the colon, uterus, and bronchi), kidney, spleen, liver and skin tissue.

One study shows that ginkgo extract helps fight PAF in asthma patients. In a double-blind trial with 8 asthmatic patients given either a standardized mixture of ginkgolides A, B and C (BN 52063), or a placebo, and were then asked to inhale allergens using an atomizer, the researchers reported that patients who took ginkgo had "significantly inhibited response to the allergens." In other words, these ginkgolides may reduce an asthmatic's bronchial constriction in response to house dust, pollen and other allergens. Ginkgo extracts may help reduce the frequency or at least the severity of asthmatic and allergic attacks. Published in 1987 (*Prostaglandins*, Vol. 34, No. 5), this study found it significantly inhibited bronchial constriction in asthmatic patients for up to six hours after they were administered the asthma-causing allergen. Several other studies have confirmed these results and also suggest a role for ginkgo biloba extract in the long-term management of asthma.

Heart-Related Disorders
When human blood cells called platelets (which help promote blood-clotting) encounter PAF, they change shape and begin to stick together. It takes only a minute quantity of PAF to cause platelets to bind irreversibly. Platelets keep us alive by stopping bleeding in emergencies, but when they stick together or "clump" on a chronic basis, they can make blood thicker and cause clotting. Platelets also secrete chemicals that cause blood vessels to constrict and cut off blood flow to vital organs. When there are excessive levels of PAF in the blood, platelets create conditions which lead to heart disease, stroke and other circulatory disorders.

In extensive tests with human blood, ginkgolides found in ginkgo extract specifically prevent PAF from binding to platelets and causing the whole range of undesirable effects mentioned above.

Eye Protection

With age, blood flow decreases to the retina, the nerve-rich area in the back of the eye necessary for sight. As the blood-starved retina deteriorates, the result is macular degeneration, a leading cause of adult blindness.

The compounds in ginkgo extract have been shown to concentrate in the eye. This, combined with ginkgo's PAF-inhibition effects, free radical and antioxidant properties and its strengthening activity on the small capillaries, ginkgo might help protect and restore healthier functioning in the eye. And indeed this is the case. In a six-month, double-blind French study of 10 people with macular degeneration, 80 mg of ginkgo taken twice a day produced "significant vision improvement."

Other studies show that ginkgo can offer protection in the cornea, as well. The cornea is the most exposed part of the eye and is open to injury and infection. One of the ginkgolide compounds in ginkgo—(ginkgolide B (BN 52021)—has been shown to inhibit PAF-mediated inflammation in the cornea, when it is applied topically on the cornea itself.

Senile macular degeneration is a growing clinical disorder in this country. This condition, which leads to a decrease in central vision and a distorted perception of the shape of objects, affects 10 percent of Americans over 65 years old. Cases in the United States are predicted to rise from 2.7 million in 1970 to over 7.5 million in the year 2030. One of the major causes is photochemical damage due to high sun exposure. It is not surprising to see a much higher incidence of macular degeneration in sunny spots like South Florida, Arizona and Southern California.

The use of antioxidant nutrients in the prevention of macular degeneration has been well-documented in the research literature. Nutrients like beta carotene (actually many carotenoids), vitamins C, E, zinc, selenium and bilberry have shown an ability to decrease the incidence of macular degeneration and, in some cases, actually slow down progression of the condition. Ginkgo biloba extract should be added to the list, as a powerful antioxidant.

A French study published in *Rokan: Recent Results in Pharmacology and Clinic* (Springer-Verlag, 1988) examines the effect of ginkgo extract on macular degeneration. This double-blind clinical study was conducted with 20 patients over 55 years of age who were diagnosed with senile maculopathy. Ten of the patients received 80 mg of ginkgo extract a day for 6 months, while the other 10 received a placebo. After 6 months of treatment, the ginkgo group showed "significant improvement" in acuity of distance vision.

The authors of this study concluded that more work needs to be done using ginkgo, but the initial results offer great hope. Thus ginkgo is well worth a try, at least as an adjunct therapy, in conditions where the function and integrity of the retina might be comprised, such as in diabetes or glaucoma.

Hearing Disorders
With age, blood flow decreases to the nerves of the inner ear. The result is cochlear deafness, a leading cause of age-related hearing loss. Hearing disorders can also be due to loud noises, atherosclerosis and cervical syndrome resulting from strain or injury to the neck—these resulting from reduction of blood circulation.

In a 30-day double-blind French study of 20 people with cochlear deafness, 80 mg of ginkgo, twice a day was compared with the standard medical therapy. The study concluded that "significant recovery was observed in both groups, but improvement was distinctly better in the ginkgo group."

Tinitus (ringing in the ears) has been observed clinically for centuries. Three factors are important in determining how successful treatment for tinnitus will be—whether the ringing is constant or intermittent; whether it is in one or both ears; and whether the ringing has been present for more than a year. If the ringing has been constant and in both ears for more than a year, the chances for a successful treatment are greatly reduced.

Several tests using ginkgo extract to treat people with tinnitus of varying degrees of severity have shown that this ailment, which is usually difficult to treat, yields nicely to ginkgo extract. For example, a 13-month study in Paris involved 103 patients with chronic tinnitus. The patients were given ginkgo biloba daily, and by the end of the trial, all participants experienced significant relief. Notably, the ringing decreased in every patient, regardless of the cause of the ringing.

In 1986, a study statistically proved the effectiveness of treatment with ginkgo extract for tinnitus; the ringing completely disappeared in 35 percent of the patients tested, with distinct improvement was seen in as little as 70 days.

One study combined chiropractic manipulation with regular doses of ginkgo extract, and it was found that this combination was more effective in restoring hearing than chiropractic manipulation alone.

In a another study, hearing weakness due to inner ear problems was treated with ginkgo extract for a period of 9 weeks. The results showed that 35 of the 59 patients in the study had either "successful" or "very successful" improvements in hearing.

Similarly, when 350 patients with hearing defects due to old age were treated with ginkgo extract, the success rate was 82 percent. Furthermore, a follow-up study of 137 of the original group of elderly patients 5 years later revealed that 67 percent still had better hearing.

Besides hearing problems, ginkgo can also be helpful for dizziness, vertigo and other equilibrium problems associated with reduced circulation in the inner ear. The combined results of 5 double-blind studies with ginkgo extract demonstrated that a daily dose of 60 to 160 mg was effective for the above symptoms in 40 to 80 percent of patients—significantly better success rate than with placebo or drugs.

Impotency

Blood flow to the penis parallels that of the heart. Impotence is a warning for developing heart disease.

Impotence is caused by arterial insufficiency and results in inability to achieve an erection, a serious problem for men. The treatment of choice is normally injections of papaverine or related drugs into the corpus cavernosum of the penis. A 1989 study reported in the *Journal of Urology* (Vol. 141) indicated that a less invasive treatment, long-term use of ginkgo biloba extract may be helpful for this dysfunction. This study, largely ignored by the media, was the first ginkgo study to appear in a U.S. medical journal.

The researchers studied ginkgo's effect on a group of 60 patients with arterial erectile dysfunction who had not responded to papaverine injections. These patients took 50 mg of ginkgo a day, for 12 to 18 months. An improvement was noted within six to eight weeks. After six months of ginkgo treatment, 50 percent of the patients had regained potency, 20 percent responded to a new trial of papaverine, 25 percent showed improved arterial inflow, but still did not respond to papaverine, and the remaining 5 percent had no clinical response. The researchers concluded: "Ginkgo appears to be very effective in the treatment of arterial erectile dysfunction." These results will hopefully lead to further research that will look into ginkgo biloba extract's effectiveness over longer periods of times.

Dosage, Safety & Toxicity

Thanks to extensive research on both humans and animals, as well as to clinical trials, the safety of long-term use of ginkgo is well understood.

The standard dose of ginkgo biloba extract is 40 mg, three times a day. The dose for a 1:1 fluid extract of ginkgo biloba is 0.5 ml three times a day. There have not been any reports of significant adverse reactions to ginkgo biloba extract at the prescribed dosages or in patients ingesting as much as 600 mg of the extract in one dose. Mild adverse reactions, though quite rare, have been reported; these include gastrointestinal upset and headache (short duration).

In one study involving 2,855 patients who took ginkgo extract, about 3.7 percent experienced minor gastric upset which had no lasting effects when the ginkgo was discontinued. Another test with 8,505 patients who took ginkgo for 6 months revealed that only 0.4 percent (33 people) experienced minor side effects, most commonly mild stomach upset.

It is noteworthy that tests show that even high doses of ginkgo extract do not change the hormonal balance in men, and that neither does ginkgo affect the sugar metabolism of the body—which means it is safe for diabetics, who often suffer from poor circulation and therefore might benefit from ginkgo treatment. Finally, no disturbances in the formation of new blood cells or the functioning of the liver and kidneys were observed, even after long-term use.

There is current on-going research showing evidence that ginkgo biloba extract may be useful as a topical cream or orally for inflammatory conditions such as sunburn, eczema, acne, psoriasis, rashes and skin allergies, and as a spray for hay fever or inflammation of the sinus cavity.

Ginkgo is not an "anti-age" remedy. But it does seem as if the wisdom locked up in each leaf of this primordial tree, ginkgo biloba, is an effective ally against many of the most harrowing symptoms of imbalance at their source. Thus while we will all get older, perhaps now we can grow old gracefully with our minds and bodies more healthfully intact.

Siberian Ginseng

The Siberian Ginseng (Eleutherococcus senticosus) is a powerful adaptogen.

As an "adaptogen," Siberian Ginseng may be without equal. The term "adaptogen" has been used in medical literature in recent years. In order to be classified as an adaptogen, a substance must meet these three following qualifications:

1. It must be non-toxic, or at least toxicity must be extremely low.

2. Its action should be nonspecific; that is, it should increase resistance to a wide variety of adverse influences, physical, chemical and biological in nature, i.e. stress, over exertion, various toxins and some infections.

3. It should possess a normalizing action. For example, a tendency to high or low blood pressure, improve circulation, increase mental alertness, concentration and memory.

According to published reports, Eleutherococcus meets all of the requirements to be classified as an adaptogen. The stem of Eleutherococcus contains a group of glycosides (eleutherosides) which possess a high biological effectiveness. The preparations from Eleutherococcus are non-toxic and harmless even when they are administered for long periods of time. These preparations improve and increase quality and quantity of physical and mental work (stimulating tonic effect). Here is what Dr. I. Brekhman wrote in his book, *Eleutherococcus*. "The capacity of Eleutherococcus to increase non-specific resistance of an organism against harmful influence of a large number of physical, chemical and biological factors (adaptogenic effect) is very important."

Siberian Ginseng has been shown to:
1. Increase physical energy, strengthen bones and tendons and aid human stamina. Tests show up to a 50 percent endurance increase in animals.
2. Increase mental alertness, accuracy and speed, improve concentration and memory.
3. Possess an anti-fatigue action that also helps motivation, coordination and resistance to stress.
4. Improve circulation as a blood pressure normalizer.
5. Stimulate carbohydrate metabolism in the liver.
6. Provide support to the endocrine system; in particular the pancreas and its action in sugar metabolism. It is reported in Japan once diabetics start on this Siberian Ginseng, the results are so favorable they never stop taking it.

Research shows that Siberian Ginseng improves sexual power, slows aging and prolongs life expectancy with use over a long period of time.

A well-known 16th century Chinese doctor once wrote, "I would rather have a handful of ginseng than a carload of gold and jewels."

GARLIC
Nature's Finest Healer

Garlic has long been used as a folk medicine. Knowledge of its effects as a tonic, invigorating agent and agent for relieving fatigue has been handed down for centuries. In the last fifty years, the medicinal properties of garlic have been studied and recognized.

The litany of therapeutic benefits of garlic is impressive. Indeed. It has been found beneficial for several diseases and conditions including high blood pressure, atherosclerosis, common cold, asthma, allergies, pneumonia, insomnia, tuberculosis, dysentery, cancer, arthritis, heart disease, diabetes, hypoglycemia and fatigue just to name a few. It has antibacterial and antifungal properties.

Scientists and nutritionists are in agreement that garlic acts as a detoxifying agent on the body; it is a powerful body cleanser. It neutralizes toxins present in the digestive tract and eliminative organs, as well as in the blood and has a beneficial effect on the function of the liver, kidneys, nervous system and circulatory system. Garlic, being an antitoxin, also strengthens the body's defenses against allergens and is, therefore, used in the treatment of allergies and asthma.

You can have all the benefits of garlic without the negative side effects of odor on your breath. The Wakunaga Company has devoted itself to the study of garlic, making incessant efforts toward eliminating the disagreeable body odor and breath and at the same time, developing the active principle of garlic into a form called Kyolic, which retains all of its best natural characteristics.

I prescribe garlic in my medical practice and receive countless positive testimonies on its effectiveness. I take it regularly and personally attest to it benefits.

SPICES[zz]

1. BLOCKS CANCER: Italian researchers recently reported in the *Journal of the National Cancer Institute* that eating rosemary, basil and parsley may cut lung cancer risk. Feeding basil leaves and cumin seeds to animals has blocked cancers, including liver cancer. At Rutgers University, applying rosemary to the skin of mice reduced the number of skin tumors by 64 percent. Herbs and spices known to have antioxidant and anti-cancer activity: rosemary, turmeric, cumin, saffron, sage, nutmeg, black pepper, thyme, ginger, cardamom, tarragon, oregano, basil and cilantro.

2. CLEANS LUNGS: Eating chili peppers is good for the lungs and helps clear stuffy noses due to colds, says Irwin Ziment, professor of medicine at UCLA. He also recommends hot peppers for emphysema, sinusitis, hay fever, asthma and chronic bronchitis. Hot foods thin secretions in the air passages: If you eat hot food, not only do your eyes water, so do your lungs. Ziment tells people with chronic breathing problems to eat three spicy meals a week. His quick decongestant: Mix 10-20 drops of hot sauce, such as *Tabasco*, into a glass of water; drink or gargle.

3. FIGHTS NAUSEA: Recent tests in Denmark showed that ginger reduced seasick sailors' vomiting by 70 percent. British research found ginger as effective as drugs at relieving nausea after surgery. To prevent motion sickness, drink tea or juice with 1/2 teaspoon ground ginger half an hour before boarding a plane or boat. The effect lasts about four hours. One study found ginger as helpful as *Dramamine*, without the side effects ie. sleepiness.

[zz] The majority of information about spices was gathered from Jean Carper's books and articles. Jean is author of *Stop Aging Now, Food Your Miracle Medicine and more.*

4. REDUCES INFLAMMATION: In Japan, an anti-inflammatory drug is based on gingerol, the aromatic compound in ginger. A study at Denmark's Odense University found that three quarters of 56 patients with rheumatoid arthritis, osteoarthritis or muscular discomfort got relief from pain and swelling after taking ginger daily for at least three months. Dose: 1/3 teaspoon ground ginger or 1 teaspoon fresh ginger root taken in food or drink three times a day.

5. THINS BLOOD: Several studies suggest ginger makes blood platelets less likely to stick together, helping to prevent blood clots that lead to heart attacks and strokes. A Danish researcher, Krishna C. Srivastava, found the same effect in cumin, turmeric and, especially, cloves, which are "stronger than aspirin in this aspect." Studies in Thailand found that eating chili peppers revved the blood's ability to dissolve clots. But the benefit lasted only 30 minutes.

6. MONITORS BLOOD SUGAR: Spices and herbs can stimulate the potency of insulin so you require less of the hormone to process sugar, says Richard Anderson of the U.S. Department of Agriculture. This could be especially important for people with Type II diabetes. Anderson's tests found sage and oregano double insulin activity; turmeric and cloves triple the activity; cinnamon is most potent. Dose: amounts common in foods. Cinnamon also may lower blood pressure, according to new research at George Washington University.

7. KILLS GERMS: Ginger and turmeric, a yellow herb used in curry powder, destroy bacteria, including salmonella, a common cause of food poisoning. Dishes such as chicken curry and ginger chicken make good health sense. Jim Duke, a medical botanist formerly with the USDA, notes that Greek fishermen cover their catch with rosemary to retard spoilage.

8. AIDS DIGESTION: Sage, dill, anise and fennel seeds help prevent intestinal gas. In a test, adding sage to cooking lentils reduced gas formation in animals dramatically. Menthol in peppermint is a smooth muscle relaxant that helps to relieve gas; peppermint oil is in many antacids, says Colin Briggs, professor of pharmacology at Canada's University of Manitoba.

9. BURNS CALORIES: In a British study, eating 3/5 teaspoon hot pepper sauce raised the metabolism 25 percent, burning an extra 45 calories in three hours. In an Australian animal test, ginger increased the metabolism 20 percent.

10. PROTECTS THE STOMACH: Several studies suggest capsaicin, the hot stuff in peppers, helps to protect the stomach by increasing mucus flow and acting as a painkiller. And research shows hot peppers and spices do not harm normal stomachs, lead to ulcers or retard the healing of ulcers. Avoid spicy foods if your stomach hurts after you eat them; spices do aggravate heartburn in some people.

EXERCISE

CONDITIONING AND AEROBICS

Since the lower extremity holds the greatest muscle mass in the body, it must be worked to achieve total body fitness.

Walking is one of the simplest forms of exercise and is a good one to start with. Whether you are walking in the park or on a treadmill, posture is very important. One of the most dramatic changes that can be made to someone's overall appearance is good posture. Creating and maintaining good posture and strengthening the necessary musculature can occur while walking. Stand tall, imagine a string pulling straight up from the center of your head. Pull your shoulders back and push your chest out. This will feel strange and uncomfortable at first, especially if you lack self-confidence. You may even feel people are looking at you, they probably are. People will notice the look of self confidence.

One more component to good posture is in hip position. It is not so much "suck your stomach in" as it is tilting your pelvis up. When your pelvis is tilted down it creates the look of a pot belly, pushing the pubis forward, pulling the hips back and squeezing the butt cheeks together will diminish any belly.

You can burn 100 calories per mile or more, if you walk up hill as you can on a treadmill. If you hold the hand rails, elevation doesn't count. Holding on counteracts any elevation you can add, test it yourself, add 15 degrees elevation and hold on for 5 minutes then try it without holding on, big difference, huh?

To get your legs in condition practice the above 3 times a week for 4 weeks, for at least 30 minutes per session, then you will be ready for the following:

Lunges	no weight,	15 reps on each leg
Deep knee bends	no weight,	20 reps
Deadlifts	25 LBS,	20 reps

One arm rows	25 LBS,	20 reps
Bench press	45 LBS,	12 reps
Military press	25 LBS,	12 reps
Skull crushers	25 LBS,	12 reps
Biceps curls	25 LBS,	12 reps
Crunches		to exhaustion

After 6 sessions do 2 sets of each exercise and after 6 more sessions do 3 sets of each exercise, the last set should be to exhaustion. Once your muscles are used to this, try a new routine eg. : Squats, Deadlifts, Pulldowns, Dumbbell bench press, Lateral raises, Triceps pulldowns, Dumbbell bicep curls, Crunches. Begin each set with a warm-up weight of 50% of your one rep max (the heaviest weight you can lift) and do 15 to 20 reps. Your second set should be 75-80% of your one rep max, do 8-12 reps. The third set should be so heavy that you can only do 4-6 reps. do this to failure (make sure you have a spotter). The last set is a cool down set. Repeat the first set.

BUILDING THE BODY—PART BY PART

Building the chest (Pectoralis major and minor)—The starting point for most chest workouts is the Bench press. This exercise concentrates on the larger, center part of the "pecs." Laying on the bench, bring the bar to your chest, then press it back up. Your hands should be spaced about one meter (one yard) apart, and the bar should always touch your chest but never bounce off it. The bar should line up with the nipples, not over the stomach or over the neck. You should not arch your back. Some people prevent arching by keeping the legs high. I don't recommend this as it makes balance more difficult. The bench press can also be done with dumbbells that allows even more range of motion and works more accessory muscles. It is a good idea to do these after regular bench press.

For travel, push-ups may be used, and a training partner can provide more weight if necessary (by sitting on your back). The push-up is virtually identical to the bench press, except upside-down.

Building the upper chest—The incline press is very similar to the bench press (which is sometimes called the "flat bench"). The only difference between the flat bench and the incline press is the body angle. If you remember that muscles can only contract to do work, you should be able to visualize how this exercise would rely more on the upper chest. Again, use full range of motion, don't arch your back, (and dumbbells are a possible alternative.) Dumbbells can be better on the incline press for people with shoulder injuries.

For travel, the "incline" or "feet up" push-up is available. You place your feet on the bed, and do pushups with your head lower than your feet.

Building the lower chest—You guessed it. Incline press for upper chest, flat bench for middle chest, and **decline press** for lower chest. Full range of motion, don't arch, and dumbbells are optional. Decline push-ups, however, are not too beneficial as there is very little body weight being lifted at this angle. An exercise called "dips" is much better. This is done with two sturdy chairs, or can be done in the gym with "dip bars." Dips are done with your elbows close to your side, your back arched, and as always, full range of motion. The third choice for lower chest is dumbbell pull-overs. Keep your butt low, and use full range of motion. Dropping the dumbbell on your face is not a good idea. Make sure any welds or bolts are secure. These pullovers also expand the rib-cage, which can give a unattractive barrel-like look to some people. If this is a problem, use one of the other exercises. Note that all of the chest exercises described so far also require the use of triceps. This is another reason why developing all muscle groups is important. Many people have difficulty developing chest muscles because the triceps muscles are too weak to allow enough weight to be used.

Building chest definition—flye motions build chest definition. The flye motion is where your arms are straight, bringing the weights from your side towards each other (in your front) until they touch. Flyes can be done with cable apparatus, or with dumbbells. Like the press exercises for building chest size, the flye exercises can build upper chest definition using incline flyes, middle chest definition using flat flyes, or lower chest definition using decline flyes. The most common mistake with flyes is to use too much weight so that the arms bend. Keep the arms straight, and use full range of motion. For travel. very wide grip push-ups are used.

Building upper back (Latisimus Dorsi "lats") —A well-built upper back, and narrow waist gives that sexy "V" shape. Although dieting for that slim waist can be a struggle, building a broad, strong upper back can be easy. The best exercise for upper back is wide grip pull-ups. The hands are placed about one meter apart, and facing away. Pull up until the bar touches behind your neck. Use both arms evenly. If the pull-up is too difficult using all your body weight, you can do the same exercise more easily as a pulldown with cable equipment. With a leg brace (or a training partner to hold you down) you can use the same cable pull-downs to actually do more than your body weight.

Building thickness to the back—Rowing motions are the opposite of pressing motions, pulling, instead of pushing. Bent over rows described here develop thickness to the back. Bend at the waist, and slowly pull the bar from the floor to your chest (and then back down). This same motion can be done with dumbbells or with cables as a cable row. Pulling the bar or cable towards the upper body (chest) develops upper back thickness. Pulling the bar or cable towards the lower body (stomach) develops lower back thickness. When in doubt as to how much weight to use, use lighter weights to prevent lower back injury. When traveling, the row motion can be done with a portable chin-bar by lying on the floor, and pulling your body up to the bar. Full range of motion is especially important when your hands are closest to your body. Pull it all the way into the body. Use smooth, controlled motions. Don't jerk.

Building lower back—Lower back size has little effect on how hot and sexy your body looks. Lower back strength does make a big difference on your chances for back injuries, for both weight training and for normal daily activities. The exercises are easy. The first choice is hyperextensions. In a gym, there is a piece of equipment called the "hyper-bench." Place yourself so that your feet are hooked under the brace, and your body is resting over the main support. Adjust this so you can freely bend at the waist. You are bent over in an upside-down "L" position, then straighten your body (using your lower back) so that you are horizontal. Slowly let your head and body go back down to the "L" position. Use full range of motion without swinging. Arch your back (and tense your back) at the top of each repetition. Keep your hands locked behind your head, or hold a weight on your chest for greater intensity. Maximum effort occurs when your back and waist are straight. For travel, use part of this same motion by just arching on the floor (optionally with a training partner holding your feet to the floor).

The next choice for lower back is called "Good mornings." With this exercise, maximum effort occurs when your waist is bent. From a standing position, bend at the waist, as low as you can go. For proper form keep your back straight, and bend only at the waist. For more resistance, good mornings can be done with a weight resting on the back of your neck.

Building arm biceps—The starting point for building biceps is the standing arm curl. This exercise is probably the easiest to do properly, but unfortunately, this is the exercise most often done improperly. Simply stand straight (and still,) holding a barbell and lift the barbell to your chest, then slowly lower it down completely. Do not "throw it," or use your back, and don't stop halfway down. Leaning against the wall with your butt and back touching is a good way to learn proper form. Also keep your elbows near your side. (Not out like chicken wings). Using a special "easy-curl" type bar allows you to do arm curls with less (unwanted) wrist strain. The results are essentially the same.

The second exercise for biceps is the preacher curl. Use a bench called a preacher or Scott bench, where the arm is supported at a specific angle. This helps reduce "cheating" and changes the hardest part of the motion to an angle different from standing. With the standing arm curl the hardest part is with your arm at 90 degrees, with the preacher curl, the hardest part is 135 degrees (with the arm not as bent). This change in angle develops a different part of the bicep. The way to avoid cheating is to keep your arm flat on the bench, don't rock back and forth. The rest of your body should be still as a rock.

Many people prefer dumbbells to help reduce cheating by reducing the total weight lifted, each arm individually uses about half the weight so that there is less of a tendency to use your back.

With care, a regular flat bench can simulate a preacher curl bench, remember to keep your body and arm still. Use the flat bench as a brace to keep your arm at a 45 degree angle, instead of hanging straight down.

When traveling, many variations of the basic arm curl motion are possible. If you don't have a chin bar, the palm toward the doorknob curl (pulling yourself on the doorknob of an open sturdy door) can be done with one or both arms. Pull up with one arm while pushing down with the other if you are truly stranded. Still try for full range of motion.

Dumbbells are used for the concentration curl. It is called the concentration curl for two reasons: One, it concentrates development in the upper bicep, and two, it requires intense concentration to do it properly. You use your own leg as a brace, instead of a piece of equipment. Concentrate on keeping your arm straight and still except for the elbow, the upper part of your arm shouldn't move. Use full range of motion. Using your leg can help keep you from cheating. Using your leg is another way to simulate a preacher curl by supporting the arm at an angle.

Developing the triceps—The triceps are three closely grouped muscles that are used to straighten the arm, the opposite of the biceps which curl the arm. Many exercises for chest can be slightly modified to exercise the triceps. Bench press becomes "close grip bench press," and for travel, push-ups become "close grip push-ups." Putting your hands at three different angles, straight, 45 degrees (inward), and 90 degrees inward, individually works each part of the triceps. Reduce intensity by moving higher, and higher (Just like push-ups for the chest). Barbell/dumbbell extensions can be visualized as the opposite of arm curls. The triceps are shortening to lift the bar, instead of the biceps shortening to lift the bar. Barbell/dumbbell extensions can be done standing or lying flat. The weight goes behind your neck. To avoid cheating, especially when standing, keep your entire body and arm still except for the elbow joint. A mirror is the best way to practice good form. Use your other hand to feel the location of the arm, don't use it to hold the arm in place.

Finally, the best way overall to develop triceps is with the cable pushdown, also called cable triceps extension. Stand close to the cable, and use full range of motion. A bent bar will reduce wrist strain without altering the results. Using narrow, medium, and wide grip will emphasize the individual parts of the triceps. Most cheating is caused by bending over as if pushing a plunger. If you feel this exercise using your shoulders, the plunger like action is the mistake. Reduce the weight until you can do it properly without bending over, and without moving your elbows from your side.

Building the forearms—Most people naturally build good forearms from gripping weights while exercising other body parts. Forearms are involved in gripping and squeezing, so the first forearm exercise is simply gripping or squeezing. Hand grips or a tennis ball provide resistance to work against. An alternate exercise is wrist curls using a barbell. The bar is let down until it is just barely held in the finger tips, and then is curled up as high as possible. Use full range of motion. Reverse curl with palms facing down, also work forearms.

Developing the shoulders (deltoids, "delts") —The best exercise for building shoulders is the lateral side raise. Pick up two dumbbells. Stand tall. Keep your arms straight and raise the dumbbells sideways to shoulder level and back down. The most important part of the shoulders to work is the middle delts. This is what gives you the broad shoulder look. To best isolate the middle delts, tip the ends of the dumbbells down as you raise them to shoulder level. It is as if they were coke bottles and you are pouring them out as you raise them up. You can have the weights slightly to the front or to the side, for the down position.

When traveling, elastic straps can provide the resistance if weights are not available. The resistance should be even throughout the lifting and the lowering motions.

Cable side raises are an added exercise that provides greater resistance at the lower part of the motion. The bent over side raise emphasizes the rear delts, and can be done standing or seated. This is the same as the lateral side raise, except that you bend over at the waist so your torso is parallel to the ground. The common error to avoid, is lifting the weights back instead of to the side. When the weights are lifted to the back the lats are being used instead of the rear delts. When seated, there is a tendency to cheat by not staying bent forward. An alternate or sometimes a supplement to the bent over side raise, is called P.O.B.N's, for Press Off the Back of the Neck. The name is self-explanatory, and full range of motion is important. Doing a head stand and pushing up is substitute for POBN's when traveling. Only for the real jock, however, they require exceptional balance, or a wall to keep you from falling over.

Building the trapezius or "traps"—may require extra effort in some people. Usually the lateral side raise and the POBN's alone are enough. If the traps are a problem area, the upright row works very well. Using either cables or barbell, with a narrow grip, raise the bar to your chin and then lower it. Keep the bar in close to your body, don't hold it away. If you are using a cable, don't step back.

Building the neck—A large neck adds to that stocky and powerful "Don't-mess-with- me" look. It can also make it very difficult to find good dress shirts. I don't recommend it. My neck size went from 15 to 16½ without doing special neck work. I include this here just for completeness.

The classic exercise is the wrestlers bridge. Supported on your feet and head (in an arch,) slowly rock side-to-side, then front- to-back. This should be done both facing up and facing down. Like the wrestlers bridge, working the neck with a training partner requires resistance up, down, and side-to-side. Unlike bridging, a training partner can help control the amount of resistance. By the way, the many straps and machines I have seen for the neck seem to take more time and effort to adjust than they're worth.

Building the thighs—There is no exercise quite like squats for building the thighs. There is also no exercise that causes more back injuries. So be warned, and start with a very, very, light weight and increase the amount slowly. **Good form is critical**. For the first few days, use a bar or broomstick with no weight at all. First, place your feet at shoulder width, pointing out slightly. Second, look high with your eyes. Pick a point up on the wall or ceiling to stare at. This will help keep your head up, and back straight. Finally, do a sitting motion, and then raise back up. A regular squat goes until your legs are parallel to the floor. A deep squat is preferred (if you have good knees) for better development, and to build and tighten the butt. The deep squat is all the way down. Front squats work the butt even more, and require careful balance. Only experienced bodybuilders should use this exercise. A tight weight belt can reduce the risk of injury for both regular and front squats. The leg press machine can also reduce this risk if you hold yourself firmly and completely seated.

In addition to the squats or leg press, you may choose to add leg extensions to build the thighs from another angle. Use full range of motion, and don't bounce. There are many travel or home exercises for the thigh. Squats can be done with your own body weight or with the extra weight of elastic straps. And step-up, step-down or climbing stairs can build your thighs. Improvise. Put your back flat against the wall and bend your knees as if sitting in a chair. Bend at exact right angles, so that your body is in the same position as if you were sitting in a chair. Hold this position for as long as possible. (At least 30 seconds.)

Lunges don't require any equipment, and some people add them to a gym routine using either dumbbells in hand or a barbell across the shoulders. From a standing position, step forward with one leg as far as you can. Keep your back knee as straight as you can. Don't let the front knee go in front of your toes. Go low enough so your thigh is parallel to the floor. Do both legs. To increase the resistance, simply hold dumbbells in both hands, or you can place a barbell on the back of your neck. Watch your lower back, keep your upper body straight and balance with the barbell.

Building the gluteus maximus ("Glutes"or Buns) Building muscle in this area creates the illusion of tight firmness. Excess fat and skin are stretched over the muscle, and as the muscles get larger, the fat becomes a smaller, less noticeable percentage. To get rid of that soft, flabby, sloppy feeling, don't worry about actual size (or on spot reducing fat) work on building firmness. Deep squats work the butt for those who can do them, and are usually adequate alone. If you can't do deep squats, there are two reasonable substitutes that can be done in the gym, at home, or traveling. Arching, while consciously tightening the buns can be done with or without extra weight and with or without a partner. Arching also helps lower back. Hyperextensions in the gym work lower back intensely and are preferred for this for efficiency reasons. Bridging is simply upside down variation of arching, with or without weight. Soft, flabby buns don't look good, or feel good.

Building the hamstrings (leg bicep)—People notice things in front of them. Because of this, arm biceps and quadriceps are often over-developed, and triceps and leg biceps are often ignored. If everyone knew how much better balanced development looks and how much easier it makes it to look good, this mistake could be avoided. Build all muscles and don't forget the hamstrings.

The best exercise is the **Straight-leg deadlift**. The deadlift uses a straight back for proper form. Do not lock your knees, keep them slightly bent. Keeping your back and legs straight, pick up the bar from the floor, and **slowly** straighten up. (Then lower it back down). The deadlift tends to keep a more constant effort throughout the entire range of motion. Another good hamstring exercise is the leg curl. There is a machine designed just for this exercise, the leg curl machine. Doing the leg curl is easy, just don't cheat by lifting off the bench or stopping halfway up. Another common way people cheat without even knowing it is to contract the calves. The gastrocnemius muscle is the outer calf muscle that give the calf it's sexy shape in women. This muscle crosses the knee and will take the resistance off the hamstrings. So, point your toes when doing these.

Another way to build the hams is with a cable machine or elastic bands. Tie an elastic band on the doorknob of a closed door and hook it around the back of your ankle. Get on the floor, on all fours and lift one leg up. With your thigh staying parallel to the floor pull the elastic strap and your foot toward your butt. While you lay on your stomach, a training partner can provide similar resistance by pushing down as you slowly "curl" each leg.

Building the calves—Running or walking on soft sand is an easy way to build calves on vacation. All other calf exercises are variations on the calf raise. Stand on a step with only the ball of your foot. Raise yourself up then completely down. The resistance is provided by your body weight. Instead of the stairway you can use a block of wood, or a special piece of gym equipment. The resistance can be increased by doing one leg at a time or by holding a dumbbell. By doing some sets with toes in, some with toes out, and some with toes forward, you exercise the entire muscle, making it grow faster.

Building the abdominals—Creating the "six pack", those abdominal ripples. Building strength and muscle in the abdominal area will help hold in that bulge. For those of you who insist on self-torture, continue doing hundreds and hundreds of sit-ups. Just please bend your knees so you don't hurt your lower back. If you want to work efficiently, however, give up those gym class sit-ups and chose one of these variations: First is the slow sit-down. Although it looks like a sit-up, it **really** works. You only have to do four to eight per set for four to six sets. Sit-up, blow out all the air and flatten your stomach. (Suck it in.) Arch your back, then, and only then, lean back slowly. Blowing out the air and arching your back makes this sit-down work all of the abdominals, not just the upper part like most sit-ups (or crunches) do. Lastly, there's the secret sit-up. Bodybuilders and the armed-forces call it the "vacuum." You can do it on the bus, in the middle of a boring meeting, almost anywhere. Slowly let out all your air so that no one notices. Then start holding in your stomach muscles tighter and tighter for as long as you can. Concentrate on doing the **lower** portion of the abs, otherwise it is too easy to do the upper part only, and forget the rest. The secret sit-up. Do it anywhere. Do it now!

That's it for all the body parts. Pick the exercises you like and that you have the equipment for. When you've done that, it's time to put together a workout schedule.

Time schedule

You already know that each muscle needs a day of rest, but there are many other considerations in choosing a schedule. For beginners three days a week are fine. After about six months you will plateau and gains will slow or stop, then you should go to a four day a week schedule. Three days per week, is OK to maintain what you have built. If you want to gain more muscle, then three days a week is not ideal because you must exercise all muscles each workout, at the end of the workout you'll be too tired to overload the muscles enough to make them grow. At four days each week, your bodybuilding chances are much better. Divide the body parts into two groups and workout half one day, and half the next. Most people do best on a Monday, Tuesday, Wednesday, Thursday routine. This matches well with the usual work week, and allows for Friday as a catch-up day for any missed workouts.

There are three basic ways of dividing the body parts into workouts Four day routine number one—upper body vs. lower body. Day one consists of exercises for the entire upper body including chest; upper and lower back; shoulders, biceps, triceps, and forearms. Day two consists of exercises for the lower body including quadriceps, butt, hamstrings, calves, and abdominals.

Another, four day routine is push motions vs. pull motions. Day one consists of exercises for muscles involved in push motions including chest, triceps, shoulders, quadriceps, butt, and calves.

Day two consists of exercises for pulling muscles such as upper and lower back, biceps, forearms, hamstrings, and abdominals. On any of these routines, always go to the next workout. Don't have Monday be day one, Tuesday day two, Wednesday day one, and Thursday day two. Most people start avoiding their least favorite workout by consistently missing Tuesdays, for example. If the last workout you did was a day one workout, the next time you workout, always do a day two workout, no matter how many days have passed. Don't cheat, and still expect to get good results.

The true bodybuilder routine—the three day split. The vast majority of successful bodybuilders split the body into three muscles groups, allowing a more intense workout for each muscle, and also allowing two days of rest for each muscle group. The standard split goes like this: Day one—Chest, upper back and lower back. Day two—shoulders, biceps, triceps, forearms. Day three—quadriceps, hamstring, glutes, calves, and abs. Notice that chest come before triceps and that back comes before biceps. If this were reversed, the exhausted triceps would limit the bench press weight so that the chest wouldn't be able to get enough overload to grow. Similarly, exhausted biceps would ruin the back workout. But since chest or back are used very little when doing triceps or biceps, doing chest and back first causes no problems when doing arms the next day.

When doing the bodybuilder routine, you can workout five or six times per week. Just remember that you always go to the next day's workout. If you are doing the day two workout, the next workout will be day three; and after day three, the next workout will be day one.

One final note on designing your program, put the heavier weight, larger muscle exercises at the beginning of each day's routine. This way, as you get more fatigued during your workout, the smaller, lighter weight exercises can still be done to the necessary overload level needed to build the muscle. For example, flye motions for chest are usually done **after** all of the heavier press motions. Schedule your energy wisely. This summarizes the basics of bodybuilding and explains how to design your program to match your goals and schedule.

Fine tuning

1. Five to ten minutes of low intensity aerobics is a good body warm up. **2.** Always warm up a body part before really working it eg.: 15 - 20 reps done with half your one rep max. **3.** Breathe, don't worry how just do it. **4.** Use free weight whenever you can they are vastly superior to machines, particularly the *Soloflex* type machines. The spring loaded "soloflex" type equipment not only suffers from lack of isolation similar to the nautilus type and piston type, but also provides very uneven resistance. The resistance is very light at the start position, and increases undesirably the further you lift or push. This uneven resistance makes it difficult to properly develop the muscle throughout the full range of motion. The people you see in their ads are built with free weights. **5.** How do I pick the best gym? Go to the gym when you would normally workout and see if is the environment you want to workout in, can you get to the equipment, or is it too crowded? Buy a one week membership to try it out. Don't be pushed into a long term contract until you know you can workout effectively. **6.** Get a training partner, not only will a partner give you incentive to show up, but your partner can spot you and help inspire you to workout harder. **7.** Studies have shown that increased sexual activity raises the level of a man's natural anabolic steroid. This steroid, which is normally provided in your body helps the muscles with protein utilization, strength, and size. Raise your body's natural steroid level, have a lot of safe sex. **8.** Get plenty of sleep, the body does most of it's healing and building during sleep. **9.** The mind is your most powerful ally, use visualization and the other techniques taught throughout this book.

The trick to establishing new habits like working out, is to break-up any old habit patterns. Do everything at once. Change all of your habits at once. Stop smoking. Stop drinking. Start working out. Diet properly. Get to sleep at a reasonable hour. Do it now, and if you miss a day or two, do it again. It takes twenty-one continuous days to get rid of bad habits and to keep new ones. Commit to twenty-one days then it will be possible. If you slip up don't beat yourself up, forgive yourself and re-commit. Start over with day one. The first 21 days are the hardest until the new habit patterns are established. Habits are a thinking shortcut that saves mental energy, but until the new habits are in place, you are going to have to think out every move. After the new habits are established, it will be harder to do something wrong! Build new habits and change your life.

So that's it. Whatever program you design, wherever you workout, and however often you workout, **the most important factor for success is persistence and consistency. Do it, Do it now, and Do it regularly. Look good, feel good, and good luck!**
Another hint to bring us to a new section—
10. Eat a healthy diet:

DIET

FOODS TO HEAL AND REJUVENATE THE BODY

- 5 - 10 servings of vegetables with one being cruciferous (broccoli, cauliflower, cabbage etc.).
- 5 or more servings of fruit (eaten between meals, not with other foods) one tomato or equivalent (tomato juice or sundried tomatoes).
- 1 serving of a legume (beans, peas, lentils or tofu).
- Bulk of calories should come from whole grains.
- Avoid all fats and oils except unrefined cold pressed oils such as: Olive oil (extra virgin) for cooking or dipping bread in.
- 4 Tablespoons of Fortified Flax or home ground flax seed (do not heat either one hotter than boiling water).
- Replace dairy (including non-fat dairy) with nut milk or low fat soy milk.
- Avoid: all meat, canned foods, processed foods especially those with partially hydrogenated oils. Meat can be replaced with 3 servings per week of deep sea fish (poached or grilled, never battered or breaded). If you absolutely must eat meat make it skinless chicken or turkey.
- Eat 9 or more small meals per day.

♥ The Five Healthy Food Groups ♥

1. **Seeds and nuts**
2. **Legumes**
3. **Fruit (including tomatoes)**
4. **Vegetables**
5. **Grains**

RECIPES

Health Elixir

1/3 package lite tofu (*Mori-Nu*®)
1 cup fresh squeezed fruit juice or nutmilk
1 Tbs. Omega Fortified Flax™
1-2 tsp. Super All Bee Power™ (*Y.S. Bee Farms*)
2 capsules Acidophilasé™ (empty the capsules)
1/2 - 1 cup frozen fruit

Directions: Add enough juice to blend tofu to creamy texture. Add remaining ingredients and blend.

Nutmilk

1/2 cup raw almonds*
6 walnut halves
2 Brazil nuts
2 Tbs. *Omega Fortified Flax*™
1 tsp. slippery elm powder
1 tsp. lecithin
1/2 package lite tofu (*Mori-Nu*®)
4-8 cups of pure water

Grind nuts in blender, add 1 cup water and blend for 1 minute. Add the rest of the ingredients and blend for 1 more minute. Add remaining water to desired thickness.

*Soaking the almonds over night greatly increases their nutritional value.

SOUPER SOUP[aaa]

1 qt. pasta sauce (non-fat or with olive oil)
2-4 cups cooked or canned beans
1 cup barley or brown/wild rice
2-4 cups fresh or frozen vegetables
3/4 cup textured vegetable protein (TVP)
1-2 cups fresh or stewed tomatoes
1 minced onion
2 celery stalks sliced
1 cup fresh or frozen spinach
4 or more cloves of garlic minced
2 Tbs. ground flax seed

Spices
2 tsp. Worchestershire sauce
2-4 bay leaves
1/2 tsp. dry mustard
1 tsp. turmeric
1 tsp. fresh ground pepper
1 tsp. curry

Optional
Sliced potatoes
Whole grain pasta

I like to start with 15 bean soup, soak over night, throw them in the crock pot on low in the morning and add the rest of the ingredients when I get home from work. I let it cook for 20 + minutes and then serve.

[aaa] This recipie contains all 5 healthy food groups.

Eggless Salad

1 10.5 oz pkg. **Mori-Nu® Silken
Lite Tofu (Extra Firm),** drained
1/2 tsp. turmeric
2 Tbs. celery, diced
1 tsp. apple cider vinegar
2 Tbs. onion, diced
2 tsp. prepared yellow mustard
1 tsp. parsley, chopped
1/2 scant tsp. white pepper
Dash paprika
1 tsp. honey

1. Crumble tofu into small mixing bowl. Set aside.
2. In a separate bowl, combine vinegar, mustard, honey and turmeric. Mix thoroughly and pour over crumbled tofu.
3. Add celery, onion, parsley, paprika and pepper. Mix thoroughly.
4. Refrigerate approximately 30 minutes to allow flavors to blend.

Note: Try Eggless Salad in a pita bread lined with fresh sprouts, lettuce or other greens.

Makes 3 servings of 1/2 cup each. Per serving: 57 calories, 1.3 g fat, 6 g protein, 131 mg sodium, 0 mg cholesterol.

Vegetable Stir Fry

3 Tbs. Sesame oil (Spectrum Naturals™)

1 pkg. Mori-Nu® (extra firm), lite Tofu cubed
2 lrg. cloves garlic, minced
2 Tbs. fresh ginger, grated
2 Tbs. lite tamari
1/2 cup green onion, chopped
6 cups of fresh vegetables (broccoli, red pepper, mushrooms, carrots, celery, snow peas, etc.)

1. Sauté garlic, ginger and tofu in oil until lightly browned.
2. Add remaining ingredients and stir fry until tender-crisp.
3. Serve over hot brown rice.

High Energy Drink

To whip up a nutritional shake, just throw the following ingredients into a blender and blend at high speed for a minute or two.

3/4 cup fresh fruit juice

1 Tbs. Omega Fortified Flax™

1 Tbs. Spectrum Naturals™ Veg
Organic Flax Seed Oil

1/2 banana (frozen)

1/3 pkg. Mori-Nu® lite tofu

Dash of cinnamon to taste

Maple syrup to taste

1 tsp. Super All Bee Power™ - (a combination of Royal Jelly, Bee Pollen, Propolis and Herbs in a powder form made from Y.S. Bee Farms).

All these items listed above are available at your health food store.

References

Reversing the Aging Process:

1. Passwater, Richard A. Ph.D. "The New Super Antioxidant Plus"
2. "Natural Health" May/June 1995.
3. Cooper, Kenneth H. M.D. "Antioxidant Revolution" as quoted in "The Saturday Evening Post" Nov/Dec 1994.
4. Baracco et al., "Gaz. Med. de France" 1981, 88:2035.
5. Carper, Jean. *Stop Aging Now* . New York: Harper Collins, 1995
6. Dartenus et al., "Bordeau Med." 13:903, 1980; Beylot et al., "Gaz. Med. de France" 87:2929, 1980; Biard et al., "Medicine Pract." 786:62, 1980; Laparra et al., "Expertise Pharmacologique" 1987.
7. "The Saturday Evening Post" Nov/Dec 1994.
8. Scambia et al., "Quercetin potentiates the effect of adriamycin in a multidrug-resistant MCF-7 human breast-cancer cell line: P-glycoprotein as a possible target" *Cancer-Chemother-Pharmacol* 1994, 34(6):459-64.
9. Yoshida et al., "The effect of quercetin on cell cycle progression and growth of human gastric cancer cells" *FEBS-Lett* Jan 15, 1990,260(1):10-3.
10. Wei et al., "Induction of apoptosis by quercetin: involvement of heatshock protein" *Cancer-Res.* Sept 15, 1994, 54(18):4952-7.
11. Rozenfel'd et al., "The possibilities of protection against local radiation injuries in ORL-oncologic patients" *Vestn-Otorinolaringol* 1990 Mar-Apr (2):56-8.
12. Timofeev et al., "The use of a solution of quercetin for the treatment of inflammatory diseases of the parotid glands" *Klin-Khir*1990 (12):20-2.
13. Galvez et al., "Antidiarrhoeic activity of quercitrin in mice and rats" *J-Pharm-Pharmacol* Feb 1993, 45(2):157-9.
14. Galvez et al "Antidiarrhoeic activity of Euphorbia hirta extract and isolation of an active flavonoid constituent", *Planta-Med.* Aug 1993, 59(4):333-6.
15. Ohnishi et al., "Quercetin potentiates TNF-induced antiviral activity " *Antiviral-Res.* Dec 1993, 22(4):327-31.
16. Mantioxidants et al., "Inhibition of aldose reductase by Chinese herbalmedicine" *Yantioxidants-Tsa-Chih* Oct 1993, 18(10):623-4, 640.
17. Hertog et al., "Dietary antioxidant flavonoids and risk of coronary heart disease: the Zutphen Elderly Study" *Lancet* Oct 23, 1993,342(8878):1007-11.
18. Gaspar et al., "On the mechanisms of genotoxicity and metabolism of quercetin" *Mutagenesis* Sept 1994, 9(5):445-9.
19. Galley et al., "A double-blind, placebo-controlled trial of a new veno-activeflavonoid fraction (S 5682) in the treatment of symptomatic capillary fragility" *Int-Angiol* Mar 1993, 12(1):69-72.
20. Galati et al., "Biological effects of hesperidin, a citrus flavonoid. (Note I):antiinflammatory and analgesic activity" *Farmaco* Nov1994, 40(11):709-12.
21. Martin et al., "Antiulcer effect of naringin on gastric lesions induced by ethanol in rats" *Pharmacology* Sep 1994, 49(3):144-50.

22. Guengerich et al., &In vitro inhibition of dihydropyridine oxidation andaflatoxin B1 activation in human liver microsomes by naringenin and other flavonoidsΔ *Carcinogenesis* Dec 1990, 11(12):2275-9.
23. Chen et al., &Flavonoidsas superoxide scavengers and antioxidantsΔ *Free-Radic-Biol-Med.* 1990, 9(1):19-21.
24. Perez-Guerrero et al., &Prevention by rutin of gastric lesions induced by ethanol in rats: role of endogenous prostaglandinsΔ *Gen-Pharmacol* May 1994, 25(3):575-80.
25. Steele et al., &Inhibition of transformationin cultured rat tracheal epithelial cells by potential chemopreventive agentsΔ *Cancer-Res* Apr 1, 1990, 50(7):2068-74.
26. Agarwal et al., &Inhibitory effect of silymarin, an anti-hepatotoxic flavonoid,on 12-O-tetradecanoylphorbol-13-acetate-induced epidermal ornithine decarboxylase activity and mRNA in SENCAR miceΔ *Carcinogenesis* Jun 1994, 15(6):1099-103.
27. &The antioxidant controversy. Grape seed extract orPycnogenol-which should you take?Δ James, &Muscle & FitnessMagazineΔ May 1995.
28. Tixier et al., Evidence by IN VIVO and IN VITRO Studies that Binding of Pycnogenols to Elastin affects its rate of Degradation of D lastases *Biochemical Phamacology* 1983, 33:24.
29. J. Masquelier, Test of capillary resistance and improved function under the influence of pycnogenol 1965.
30. Hertog et al., Intake of potentially anticarcinogenic flavonoids and their determinants in adults in the Netherlands *Nutr-Cancer* 1993, 20(1):21-9.
31. Planta Medica, 43:101-120, 318-22, 1981 Am J. Chin. Med., 7:197-236, 1979 Biochem. Pharm., 33:3491-7, 1984
32. Herbal Medicine, Gothenburg, Sweden: AB Arcanum, pp. 162-69.

Glucosamine:

1. J.S. Lawrence, &Rheumatism in PopulationsΔ. Heinemann Medical (1977), London.
2. R.R. Vidal y Plana, K. Karzel, Pharmacol Res Comm 1978; 10: 557. L.S. McKenzie, B.A. Horsburgh, P. Ghosh, T.K. Taylor, Lancet 1976, 1:908.
3. K. Karzel, R. Domenjoz, Pharmacology 1971; 5: 337.
4. See references 2 and 5.
5. G. Crolle, E. D Este, Curr Med Res Opin 1980; 7: 104-109.
6. J.M. Pujalte, E.P. Llavore, F.R. Ylescupidez, Curr Med Res Opin 1980; 7: 110-114.
7. A.L. Vaz, Curr Med Res Opin 1982; 8: 145-149.
8. I. Setnikar, M.A. Pacini, L. Revel, Arzneim-Forsch/Drug Res 1991; 41: 542-545. I. Setnikar, R. Cereda, M.A. Pacini, et al, Arzneim-Forsch/Drug Res 1991; 41: 157-161.
9. J. Grevenstein, I. Michiels, M. Arens-Corell, et al, Acta Orthopaedica Belgica 1991; 57: 157-161.
10. A. Reichelt, et al, Arzneimettel-Forschung 1994; 44: 75 - 80.

Tofu References

1. Librato A. Santiogo, Midori Hiramatsi, Akitane Mori. *Japanese soybean paste miso scavenges free radicals and inhibit lipid peroxidation.* J Nur Sci Vitaminol 38:297–304, 1992.
2. MR Lovati, C Manzoni, A Corsini, A Granata, R Frattini, R Fumagalli, CR Sirtori. *Low Density Lipoprotein Receptor Activity is Modulated by Soybean Globulins in Cell Structure.* J Nutr 122: 1971–8; 1992.
3. Vucenick, I., VJ Tomazic, D. Fabian, AM Shamsuddin. *Antitumor activity of phytic acid (inositol hexaphosphate) in murine transplanted and metastic fibrosarcoma, a pilot study.* Cancer Letters 65:9–13; 1992.
4. Dunn, C, Liebman, M. *Plasma Lipid Alterations in Vegetarian Males Resulting From the Substitution of Tofu for Cheese.* Nutr. Research 6:1343–1352, 1986.
5. Smith, G.D. and J. Pekkanen. *Should there be a moratorium on the use of cholesterol lowering drugs?* Brit Med J 304:431–4; 1992.
6. First International Symposium on the Role of Soy in Preventing and Treating Chronic Disease. Lectures and poster presentations, Feb. 20–23, 1994, Mesa Pavilion Hotel, Mesa, Arizona.
7. Messina, Mark Ph.D., Messina, Virginia, R.D. *The Simple Soybean and Your Health.* Avery Publishers, New York, 1994.

Suggested Reading

Physical Health

1. *Antioxidant Revolution* by Kenneth H. Cooper, M.D.
2. *Conscious Eating* by Gabriel Cousens, M.D.
3. *Diet for a New America* by John Robbins
4. *Dr. Whitaker's Guide to Natural Healing* by Julian Whitaker, M.D.
5. *Essential Fatty Acids in Health and Disease* by Edward N. Siguel, M.D., Ph.D.
6. *Fats that Heal, Fats that Kill* by Udo Erasmus
7. *Hands on Healing* by the editors of *Prevention* magazine
8. *Juicing for Life* by Cherie Calbom and Maureen Keane
9. *McDougall Plan* and more by John McDougall, M.D.
10. *Reversing Heart Disease and Eat More, Weigh Less* by Dean Ornish, M.D.
11. *Spontaneous Healing* by Andrew Weil, M.D.
12. *Staying Healthy with Nutrition* by Elson M Haas, M.D.
13. *Stop Aging Now!* and *Food Your Miracle Medicine* by Jean Carper

Cookbooks

The New McDougall Cookbook by John and Mary McDougall
The American Vegetarian Cookbook by Marilyn Diamond

Spiritual and Emotional Health

1. Books and tapes by Anthony Robbins
2. Books and tapes by Deepak Chopra. M.D.
3. Books and tapes by Denis Waitley
4. Books and tapes by Susan Smith Jones
5. *Chicken Soup for the Soul, 2nd Helping* and *3rd Serving* by Jack Canfield and Mark Victor Hansen
6. *Choose to Live Peacefully* and *Choose to Live Each Day Fully* by Susan Smith Jones, Ph.D.

7. *Closer to the Light* by Melvin Morse, M.D. and Paul Perry
8. *Discovering the Laws of Life* by Sir John Marks Templeton
9. *Facing Codependancy* by Pia Mellody and Adrea Wells Miller
10. *Healing the Shame that Binds Us* and more by John Bradshaw, Ph.D.
11. *Healing Words* by Larry Dossey, M.D.
12. *How to Talk to Anyone, Anytime, Anywhere* by Larry King
13. *How to Win Friends & Influence People* by Dale Carnegie
14. *Journey of Souls* by Michael Newton, Ph.D.
15. *Life 101* series of books by John-Roger and Peter McWilliams
16. *Love Medicine and Miracles* and *Peace, Love & Healing* by Bernie Siegel, M. D.
17. *Men Are From Mars, Women are from Venus* and more by John Gray, Ph.D.
18. *No Ordinary Moments* and *Way of the Peaceful Warrior* by Dan Millman
19. *Real Moments* and more by Barbara DeAngelis, Ph.D.
20. *Return to Love* and more by Marianne Williamson,
21. *Road Less Traveled* and more by M. Scott Peck, M.D.
22. *The Power Of Positive Thinking* and more by Norman Vincent Peale
23. *Timeless Healing* and more by Herbert Benson, M. D.
24. *You'll See It When You Believe It* and more by Wayne Dyer, Ph.D.

About the Author

Dr. Brian K. Bailey, is a Podiatric Physician & Surgeon and an Associate of the American College of Foot & Ankle Surgeons. He lectures on health-related topics throughout the United States and Canada. Brian is also a personal fitness trainer, free-lance writer, author and wellness consultant.

Beginning in 1997 Dr. Bailey plans to leave his practice of podiatric medicine to follow his own advice and follow his purpose. He now devotes his time to the advancement of human potential through his writing, lectures, workshops and personal counseling.

In order to reach more people Dr. Bailey will move from his small community in North Bend, Oregon to the Fort Lauderdale-Miami area in Florida.

Dr. Bailey will continue to travel throughout the world to deliver his message of optimal wellness of the body, mind and spirit. He also develops personalized wellness programs for individuals families and corporations.

Dr. Bailey also does consultation over the phone, mail or e-mail. To arrange lectures, workshops or counseling contact Dr. Bailey at:

HEALTH UNLIMITED
1890 Waite St. Suite 6
North Bend, OR 97459
(541) 756-3332

E-mail: DrBBailey@AOL.com
        or
102127,2171@compuserve.com